THE ❧ IRON ❧ ROSE

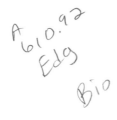

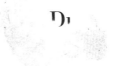

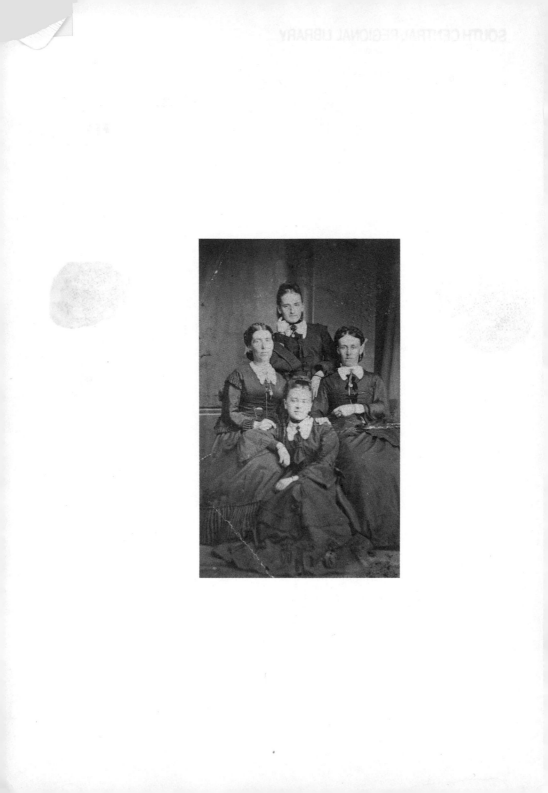

THE ❧ IRON ❧ ROSE

The Extraordinary Life of Charlotte Ross, M.D.

FRED EDGE

University of Manitoba Press

© Fred Edge 1992

Published by University of Manitoba Press
Winnipeg, Manitoba R3T 2N2

Printed in Canada

Printed on acid-free paper ∞

Design by Norman Schmidt

Frontispiece: Charlotte Ross standing at centre (courtesy Ruth Wardrop).

Cover illustration: Charlotte Ross (courtesy Ruth Wardrop).

Photographs courtesy of Phyllis Backman (4, 8, 13, 16, 17, 25, 27, 28), the
Canadian Pacific Archives (10) and Ruth Wardrop (all other photographs).

Cataloguing in Publication Data

Edge, Fred, 1927-

The iron rose

ISBN 0-88755-154-8 (bound) — ISBN 0-88755-627-2 (pbk.)

1. Ross, Charlotte, 1842-1916. 2. Physicians - Manitoba - Whitemouth -
Biography. 3. Women physicians - Manitoba - Whitemouth - Biography.
I. Title.

R464.R67E34 1992   610'.92   C91-097200-1

The publication of this volume was assisted by grants from the Canada
Council/Conseil des Arts du Canada and the Manitoba Arts Council/
Conseil des Arts du Manitoba.

*I apply the dressing,
but God heals the wound.*

Ambroise Paré (1510-1590)
Sixteenth-century pioneer in modern surgery

CONTENTS

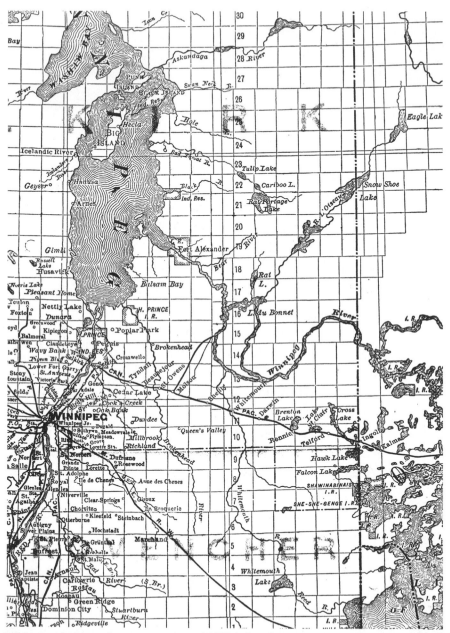

Whitemouth, Manitoba, at centre, around 1900 (taken from section map, *Descriptive Atlas of Western Canada*, published by the Minister of the Interior, 1900).

It was not until the summer of 1980 that I first heard of Charlotte Ross. My wife, Christina, and I were living on a turn-of-the-century homestead, a mile or so from a crossroads called River Hills, not far from the town of Whitemouth, Manitoba.

The Whitemouth Municipal Museum Society had published a book the previous year called *Trails to Rails to Highways*. It told the history of the region and its pioneer families, mostly based on interviews with present-day descendants, but also through old letters, diaries and family bibles. Christina's attention was caught by a brief biography of Dr. Charlotte Whitehead Ross, reprinted from a paper written for a Winnipeg reading club in 1933. She showed it to me. We agreed that Charlotte had been much too remarkable a person, her life far too consummate both personally and professionally, to remain so sketchily remembered.

We began conversations with one of Charlotte's granddaughters, then living in Lac du Bonnet, just northeast of Whitemouth, and two others in Winnipeg, about sixty-five miles to the southwest. These led to almost eight years of research involving persons and places in five provinces and four countries, all of whom had touched or been touched by Charlotte during her lifetime.

By any standards, let alone those of a socially prominent family living in British North America in the late 1800s, Charlotte was an unusual person. A century before liberated woman, she broke from her Victorian world of traditional roles and social proprieties, titled royalty and railway barons, politicians and prime ministers, to achieve her own freedoms.

When prejudice against her sex denied her entrance to medical schools in Canada, she graduated from the Woman's Medical College of Pennsylvania. When her credentials were refused, she practised unlicensed in Montreal as Quebec's first woman doctor. When her husband went to Manitoba to work with her father on the construction of the Canadian Pacific Railway, she joined him with their five children and became the first woman doctor to practise in the West. Still denied a licence, she treated the men who built the railway, and the families who followed it to their homesteads.

A devout Presbyterian, Charlotte was also remarkable for her early sense of ecumenicity. Born into a Methodist family in Yorkshire, England, she finished her general education in a Quebec convent and studied medicine at a Quaker college in Philadelphia. Her Whitemouth cabin and later the church that she and her husband built were open to Sunday services, including a wandering evangelist who called himself Father Christmas.

Daughter, wife, mother, physician and surgeon, she was a

little of Auntie Mame, a little of Mother Theresa, but always her own woman. Over more than seven years of growing to know Charlotte Ross, her family, friends, times and circumstances, I am indebted to a great many people and wonderfully human institutions.[1]

I am particularly grateful to my wife for finding Charlotte and devoting so much of her time and herself to helping research her story; to Airdrie Bell Cameron, who wrote the reading-club paper on her in 1933; to Pierre Berton, Harry J. Boyle, the late Morley Callaghan, the Canada Council and Jack McClelland for their early encouragement and support; to Michael Century and the Banff Centre for providing an evocative work-place when I needed one; to descendants of the Whitehead and Ross families for graciously sharing their time and memories;[2] and to Doris Batkin, historian, and Shirley Falconer, librarian, Clinton, Ontario, for providing the answers to so many questions.

I also wish to express my gratitude to my two consultants on religion and medicine. Dr. Bruce Miles is a former moderator of the Presbyterian Church in Canada, and served for many years as pastor of Winnipeg's First Presbyterian Church. Dr. Rognvald (Ron) Bowie is a senior staff member at the Health Sciences Centre, Winnipeg.

Finally, I wish to thank posthumously William Luxton of *The Free Press*, and Amos Rowe of *The Times*, whose lively reportage in the late 1800s proved so useful in providing much of the background to Charlotte's thirty-one years on the Manitoba frontier.

THE ❦ IRON ❦ ROSE

I have written *The Iron Rose* as a dramatized biography. I did this to breathe life into someone so full of life that any other treatment seemed inappropriate. Should I be thought presumptuous in putting words in Charlotte's mouth, they vocabularize an intimate knowledge of her character and personality, based on my understanding of the life she lived and the remarkably precise memories of her grandsons and granddaughters. Her manner of speech in this work was shaped by the same family sources, collections of Victorian letters, and by my own childhood as the son of an English immigrant and second-generation railroader, in a family not unlike the Whiteheads' and the Rosses'.

Throughout *The Iron Rose,* I have never allowed dramatic values to take precedence over factuality. My objective from start to finish has been to make this an honourable testimony to a woman whose life was eminently so. If the result makes you feel that you have somehow known and loved Charlotte Ross, as I have, then I will have succeeded.

F.E.
Leighton Artist Colony
Banff Centre
Banff, Alberta

1 Archdiocese of Toronto, Roman Catholic Church, Archives; Archives and Special Collections of Women in Medicine, Medical College of Pennsylvania and Hospital, Phildelphia; Archives des Religeuses Hospitalières

de Saint-Joseph (Hôtel Dieu), Montreal; Archives of the Sisters of Charity "Grey Nuns," Province of St. Boniface, St. Boniface, Manitoba; Canadian Medical Association, Ottawa; Canadian Railway Museum, Saint-Constant, Quebec; Centennial Library, Winnipeg; College of Physicians and Surgeons of Manitoba, Winnipeg; College of Physicians and Surgeons of Ontario, Toronto; Convent of the Sacred Heart, Montreal and Winnipeg; Corporation professionnelle des medecins du Quebec, Montreal; First Presbyterian Church, Winnipeg; Free Library of Philadelphia; Henry Birks and Sons Limited, Montreal; Public Archives of Manitoba, Winnipeg; Manitoba Legislative Library, Winnipeg; Manitoba Medical Association, Winnipeg; Manitoba Pharmaceutical Association, Winnipeg; McGill University, Montreal; Metropolitan Toronto Library; Ontario Ministry of Education, Toronto; National Railway Historical Society, Newark, Delaware, U.S.A.; Osler Library, McGill University; Public Affairs, Canadian Pacific Railway, Winnipeg; River Heights Public Library, Winnipeg; Ross United Church, Whitemouth, Manitoba; Special Collections, Bishop's University Library, Lennoxville, Quebec; St. Mary's Academy, Winnipeg; St. Mary's Cathedral, Winnipeg; Town of Clinton, Ontario; University of Manitoba, Winnipeg; University of Toronto; Ville de Montréal, Secretariat Municipal, Division des Archives; Whitemouth Municipal Museum Society, Whitemouth, Manitoba; Winnipeg School Divison No. 1.

2 Phyllis Backman, Patricia Smerchanski and Ruth Wardrop, Winnipeg; the late Dr. Donovan Ross, Fallis, Alberta; Douglas Ross, Vernon, British Columbia; Lewis Whitehead, Brandon, Manitoba; William Whitehead, Winnipeg.

Whitehead-Ross Family Tree, 1833-1888

Joseph
Whitehead
b. 1814

m. Isabella Gibbings 1832   m. Margaret McDonald 1854   m. Harriett (McKay) 1883   m. Catherine Little 1893

Charles b. 1836 — m. Hanna Lake 1861

Mary Anne b. 1841 — m. Thomas Fair 1861

Charlotte b. 1843 — m. David Ross 1861

William b. 1849 — m. Caroline Nicholson 1874

Bella b. 1862 — m. Fremont Wood 1883

Kate b. 1865 — m. P.D. McKinnon 1884

Min b. 1867 — m. Hope Ross* 1887

Carrie b. 1873

Hales b. 1875

Joseph b. 1881

Donnie b. 1883

Lottie b. 1888

* same surname, no relation

THE ❧ IRON ❧ ROSE

CHAPTER ❦ ONE

Montreal, Spring, 1869

*C*HARLOTTE STOOD IN THE FOYER of her in-laws'
country estate in Côte des Neiges, on the Tollgate Road
just north of Montreal. She finished reading the letter
from her stepmother that had arrived by that morning's post.
She leaned forward, closing her eyes. The tips of her fingers
pressed against the polished mahogany table top.

Mary Anne was dying.

Charlotte let the letter drop to the silver salver on the entry-
hall table. Her lips made a silent prayer, practising an acceptance
through faith that she had learned at an early age. Both her
Yorkshire mother, Isabella, and a younger brother, Joseph Jr.,
had died within three weeks of each other eighteen years earlier.
Charlotte had been seven. Mary Anne had been two years older.
Charlotte picked up the single page Margaret had written, and
read it again, more slowly this time.

Clinton, April 15

Dear Charlotte:
I pray this letter finds you and David and the children in good health.

It is with a heavy heart that I write to advise you that following her attack over Christmas last, which worsened into spring, little hope now is held for your sister's eventual recovery.

The weak lungs that have troubled her for so long, confining her to her bed soon after your return to Montreal, show no signs of strengthening. The exact opposite, in fact, is true.

I have written your father, who is attending the House in Ottawa, advising him of the seriousness of Mary Anne's condition. Dr. Cole is uncertain as to how much time is left to her, apparently being either a matter of weeks, or some few months, depending on His will.

Since you so well and selflessly have cared for your sister over her many illnesses, I know that you need no urging from me to come now to be by her side. As always, God bless you for this.

Margaret

Charlotte folded the page. She thoughtfully fitted it into its envelope. From her early teens, she had helped nurse Mary Anne through the recurring illness that had made her a chronic invalid. She had done this gladly, out of the closeness they had shared since the death of their mother. In time she had become practised at it, adding professional advice and home study to the practical experience she gained in her sister's sickroom.

Now she brought herself back to the present, mentally cataloguing what she must do before leaving for Clinton. First, of course, she must speak to her husband. She tucked Margaret's letter into the lace waistband of her dress. Then she went to tell the houseman to harness the horse and buggy and bring it around to the front entrance.

The family-owned wholesale house of Whitehead and Ross, with which David Ross worked as a commercial traveller, supplied stores that catered to the tastes and thirsts of well-to-do Quebeckers. It dealt in domestic and imported bottled, canned and packaged foods and spirits in case lots. For much of the time David was on the road handling the bulk buying and selling. This week he had remained in the city to catch up on his paperwork. Charlotte found him seated at his desk in a small office at the rear of the store, going over orders and invoices. He looked up as she entered, mildly surprised at the unexpected visit.

"Well, hello!" He scraped back his chair, standing.

"This came this morning," Charlotte said, taking Margaret's letter from her handbag. "It's about Mary Anne."

"Bad news?" When Charlotte did not reply, David took the letter and began reading.

"I decided to bring it," Charlotte said, "rather than wait until you got home."

David's concern showed in his deepening frown. When he had finished, he handed the letter back to Charlotte. "I'm sorry."

"It wasn't unexpected." She put the letter back in her purse. "It's been so long since she's been really well. At Christmas, remember? We both noticed."

They were silent for a moment.

"I'll have to go to Clinton right away," Charlotte said. David nodded.

"I'll take Kate and Min with me. Bella can come when she's finished school."

"Yes."

"I thought we'd leave in a day or so. It will take me that long to get packed." She paused. "I don't know how long we'll be gone. You won't mind?"

"No, I won't mind. Of course not."

"It may be for several months. I pray it will be."

David nodded. "For as long as it is, I won't mind."

Two days later Charlotte was ready to leave for Clinton with Kate, who was three, and Min. The youngest of her three daughters was eighteen months, and had been named Mary Anne Fair for her aunt. It was agreed that Bella would join her mother and two sisters after school closed for the summer holidays the last week in June, when Bella turned seven. All the family and the Rosses' housegirl left early in the morning by carriage for the Grand Trunk Railway Station in Montreal. The express to Toronto departed daily at 8:30 a.m.

While the housegirl watched over the two other children in their passenger-car seats, Bella stood with her mother and father on the station platform. Charlotte and David spoke idly, lapsing into long silences. David realized that in spirit his wife already was by her sister's side in Clinton. Finally the conductor looked at his railway watch, then up and down the length of the platform. He slipped his watch back into his waistcoat pocket and called out "All aboar-r-d!" – grandly rolling his r's, as Bella expected he would, as railway conductors always did.

"You be a good girl, now!" Charlotte stooped to give her eldest daughter a quick embrace and a kiss on the cheek.

"I will."

"You understand why I have to go, to be with your Aunt Mary Anne? She's very ill, and she needs me."

Bella nodded just a little.

"We'll celebrate your seventh birthday at Grandfather's." The housegirl rejoined them on the station platform. Charlotte straightened, brushed David's cheek with her lips, and stepped up into the railway car.

"Mother! I want to go, too!"

At Bella's sudden cry, Charlotte hesitated long enough to call out to her husband. "Speak to her, David!"

Then she was gone, inside the car, making her way down the aisle to where her two younger daughters sat. As the train jerked to a start, she bent and caught a last glimpse of Bella standing lonely by her father. One hand was bunched at her eyes, the other was waving goodbye to all the strangers in the moving windows.

The train ride from Montreal took sixteen hours, arriving in Toronto a half-hour past midnight. Whenever Charlotte travelled between Montreal and Clinton, she stopped overnight with her uncle and aunt on her stepmother's side, Senator

Donald McDonald and his wife, Frances. Although the McDonalds had fourteen children of their own, there was always plenty of room for guests. They lived in a twenty-six-room house in an exclusive neighbourhood on southeast Queen Street.

The McDonalds were fond of their attractive young niece. They saw her as an engaging slip of a woman, not five feet tall, always fashionably turned out, and looking younger than her twenty-five years. Although they would have liked her to stay another day or two, they understood her desire to get to Clinton as soon as possible.

After Charlotte and the children had managed a few hours' sleep, the McDonalds' houseman drove them to the railway station. They caught the Grand Trunk for Stratford at 7:30 a.m. They changed trains there with just enough time for luncheon before making their northbound connection at one o'clock. The line they rode for an hour and a half between Stratford and Clinton had been called the Buffalo, Brantford and Goderich Railroad before being taken over by the Grand Trunk. Built by Charlotte's father fourteen years earlier, it had made him a wealthy man.

CHAPTER TWO

Clinton, Spring, 1869

C HARLOTTE AND THE CHILDREN were met at the station by her younger brother, William. He was nineteen, in his second-year apprenticeship in Clinton with R.W. Watts and Co., Chemists and Druggists.

Charlotte loved both her brothers, almost as much as she did Mary Anne, but of the two she had a particularly warm feeling for William. She thought this was because he had been so young when all four of them had been left motherless. William had been seventeen months when their mother, at thirty-seven, and her five-year-old son had died of diphtheria. Now it was their sister, chronically ill since childhood, who was near death.

Charlotte had decided long ago that, as much as her staunch Christian upbringing allowed her to hate anything, she hated illness.

"Has Mary Anne's condition changed any?"

William had finished roping their luggage to the rear of the half-covered carriage and pair. He took the driver's seat beside Charlotte. "No." His voice, like his face, was suddenly glum. "I wish I could tell you different." He released the carriage brake and gave a quick flick of the reins. The team moved off smartly.

"Have you seen Charles lately?"

"Just last week." William's manner regained some of the animation of his original welcome. "He says the grist mill is making Father mountains of money. Not only that, but Charles has been named Blyth's first justice of the peace. Can you imagine? Our Charles a JP?" For whatever reason, William found this personally difficult. He shook his head in amused disbelief.

Their older brother was thirty-two. The same summer as her own marriage to David, and Mary Anne's to Thomas Fair, Charles had married a Smiths Falls woman named Hanna Lake. Their friends still referred to 1861 as the year of the Whitehead weddings.

"Hanna and the children are well?"

"Just fine," William said, with a grin over his shoulder at Kate and Min. "They're both looking forward to seeing their cousins again."

William deposited Charlotte and his two nieces at the front entrance to the grand new house Joseph Whitehead had built two years earlier on three scenic acres. Margaret had been awaiting their arrival at the parlour window. She embraced her stepdaughter, then stepped back with both Charlotte's hands in hers.

"I'm so glad you could come so quickly."

While William helped George, the houseman, unload the luggage and carry it into the house, Margaret fussed over the children. She exclaimed at how much they had grown, even though less than four months had passed since Christmas, when she had last seen them. She listened attentively and responded in kind to Kate's excited questions.

Yes, their grandfather still had his muster of pretty peacocks. . . . No, they couldn't visit them and the horses until they were settled in and someone went with them. . . .Yes, Bella could see the animals too, when school was out and she came to Clinton.

Charlotte's father had married Margaret McDonald three years after the deaths of his first wife and their young son. Charlotte knew about the gossip that her father had married Senator McDonald's thirty-year-old spinster sister for social and political reasons, leading to the railway-construction contract that had made him his fortune. She did not doubt that this was partly true. She also knew that whatever else Margaret had brought to her widowed father, love for him and his young family had been the most lasting part of her dowry.

Finally, Kate and Min were seated at the kitchen table with milk and sugar cookies served by Barbara, the housegirl, George's wife. Charlotte went with her stepmother into the parlour.

"Would you like a cup of tea?" Margaret asked.

"No, thank you."

"I'm so pleased you're here."

"The moment I got your letter I took it to David, and he agreed that I should leave at once. I started packing that same evening." She paused. "It's still as serious as you said in your letter?"

Her stepmother nodded slowly. "She seems to get a little better for short periods. But then the coughing starts again, with the blood. Charlotte, you'll scarcely recognize her, she's lost so much weight."

"Then there isn't much hope?"

"Dr. Cole says no."

Mary Anne's physician was an Irishman from Dublin, a graduate of prestigious University of Trinity College. He was popular with his patients, although some thought he was overworked and charitable to a fault.

"I heard back from your father," Margaret said. "There isn't anything he can do, and the House is in session. He asked to be informed at once if there's any change. He'll be thankful you've come."

Charlotte nodded. "She's had such a bad cold for so long this time. Why didn't she see the doctor sooner?"

Margaret sighed. "You know Mary Anne."

"Yes."

"Dr. Cole has been very good, as he's always been. He's been doing everything he can."

"I'm sure he could have done more, if he'd been called sooner."

"Her husband tried," Margaret said defensively. "I tried. It was Mary Anne. She kept insisting she didn't want to be a bother."

Charlotte rose. "I'm sorry. Of course you all did your best. I just wish I could have been here to help."

Margaret watched while her stepdaughter walked to the window and stood looking out. She got up and went to her,

gently placing a hand on Charlotte's arm. "You're here now."

"Yes." Charlotte covered her stepmother's hand with her own, then turned to face her. "I think I'll go to see her."

"Do. I've already told her you were coming.

"Will you ask George to get the buggy ready?"

"Yes. I'll stay and look after the children." She brightened. "I know it's only been since Christmas, but it seems like an age since I last saw them!"

From the Whiteheads', at the edge of town, it was a short ride to Thomas Fair's place on Main Street. He and his family lived in a simple frame building with the post office in front, living quarters behind, and bedrooms on the second floor.

Charlotte chose to drive her father's democrat, which the houseman hitched up and brought around to the front entrance. Joseph Whitehead's fringe-topped black buggy with the bright yellow wheels was as familiar a sight around Clinton as he was himself. He and his family were among the region's earliest settlers. Twenty years earlier, they had left England for British North America aboard a steam-assisted sailing ship. There had been no Clinton then, just a crossroads called The Corners. Active in the life of the new town, Charlotte's father had been its first reeve. Two years before, at Confederation, he had been elected to go to Ottawa as an opposition member in Sir John A. Macdonald's coalition government.

Respect for Joseph and his family was evident as Charlotte wheeled onto Main Street. Townspeople in several passing buggies nodded or tipped their hats to her; she returned these

THE 🌹 IRON 🌹 ROSE

greetings as cheerfully as her concerned state of mind permitted. She was tethering her horse to the hitching post in front of the post office when someone called her name.

"Charlotte Ross!"

She looked up at Margaret Hale.

"Are you just visiting, or here to stay a while?"

"I'm here to see Mary Anne," Charlotte said.

"I heard she's been feeling poorly these past few weeks. It's nothing serious?"

"I'm afraid yes."

"I'm sorry. I didn't know." She hesitated. "If there is anything Horatio or I can do . . ."

"It's kind of you to ask, but I'm afraid there isn't much that can be done."

"Well, do please pay us a visit, whenever you can."

"Thank you. I will."

Charlotte watched Margaret retreat up the street. The Hales were an interesting couple. Margaret was a Pugh, as old a Clinton family name as the Whiteheads' own. She had married an American. Horatio was a Harvard graduate and ethnologist from New Hampshire who divided his time between his law practice and studies of the region's Indians. He also worked with the Reverend A.K. McDonald, the Presbyterian pastor who had joined in marriage all three Whiteheads, towards improving the quality of schooling in his adopted town.

Charlotte entered the post office under the tiny bell that tinkled over the door. Her brother-in-law was sorting mail, stuffing letters into the wall of pigeonholes behind the counter. At the sound of the bell he turned. He gave Charlotte a quick smile of gratitude.

"Thank you for coming."

"How is she?"

"Not very well these last few days."

"And the children?"

"They're fine. William is too young to understand, but I think Josie does."

Charlotte nodded. Her niece, named Josephine for her grandfather Joseph, was about the same age as Bella. William Dickson Fair (both William and Dickson were family names) was no older than Kate.

Charlotte saw that her brother-in-law was feeling the strain of the previous few months.

"I've come to do what I can to help," she said.

"I know. Margaret told Mary Anne you were coming. She's been looking forward to it."

Charlotte walked behind the counter and placed a hand on her brother-in-law's arm. The gesture moved him to sudden anguish.

"My God, Charlotte, she's only twenty-eight."

Charlotte looked into Thomas's eyes and felt a well of sympathy for what she saw there. He turned away not speaking, and she wondered what he might want to say to her. That Mary Anne's life, hardly begun, was already coming to an end? That this was cruel and unjust to him and the children? Every Sunday,

Charlotte and her sister and brothers had sat in the parlour while first their mother, then Margaret, had read aloud from the family Bible. "In this as in all things," she remembered from her childhood of Sundays, "let God's will be done."

"I'll go and see her now," Charlotte said.

She walked around the counter to the door that led to the rear and the stairway upstairs. When she turned at the bottom of the stairs, Thomas still had his back to her. "It's hard for me," she said. "Please believe I understand how much harder it is for you and the children." It was all she could give him.

Mary Anne was lying in bed, propped up by pillows, her eyes closed as though she were sleeping. As much as Charlotte had prepared herself for what her long illness had done to Mary Anne, she was shocked by her sister's appearance. She was pale and thin, her cheekbones much too pronounced, her arms frail and white above the covers. Charlotte hesitated, then spoke in just a whisper. "Are you awake?"

Mary Anne opened her eyes and gave her sister a weak smile. "Lately, I'm never quite sure."

Charlotte smiled back. "I've come to look after you. I'm going to stay right by your side until you're up and around again."

Mary Anne did not reply. She tried to work herself up into more of a sitting position, and Charlotte leaned forward to help.

"You always did like to play nursemaid," Mary Anne said. "Remember the day in the barn when the swallow fell out of its nest?"

Charlotte laughed at the recollection.

16

"And the mother swallow kept swooping down on you because you had her baby!" she said.

"You made me hold it so none of the cats could get it," said Mary Anne.

"I had to get the ladder."

"Yes, but I was the one the mother swallow was mad at. I thought she'd peck my eyes!"

"Well, anyway, it all worked out."

Mary Anne chuckled. "When Father caught you up that rickety old ladder, you almost got a good lickin'."

"I had to put the baby back in its nest."

"Yes, but Father was afraid you'd fall and hurt yourself."

"I almost did!"

Mary Anne started to laugh, but the laugh became a cough that shook her whole body. Finally it subsided and she fell back exhausted against the pillows. Charlotte picked up the ironstone washbowl from the table by Mary Anne's bed and held it to her chin. She frowned at the flecks of blood in the mucus her sister spat into the basin.

Mary Anne caught Charlotte's frown as she put the washbowl back on the bedside table.

"I'm sorry," said Mary Anne.

"For what?"

"For being such a bother."

"Don't be a silly goose."

Mary Anne nodded towards the washbowl. "It's not very pleasant, I know."

"Being sick isn't pleasant," said Charlotte. "But you 'll get better."

"I don't think so."

Charlotte saw something in her sister's eyes she had never seen before. It puzzled her because it was a darkly intangible yet growing presence, like a shadow that lengthens into evening and disappears in darkness. She wondered if it was fear. Of what? Of suffering? Of dying? Of what comes after death? Sitting by her sister, wanting to reach out across the intimacies and experiences they had shared from childhood, Charlotte realized that in this way at least they were strangers. Mary Anne already was someplace she had never been.

"I have to go now," Charlotte said.

Mary Anne took hold of her sister's hand. "You 'll come back soon? Tomorrow? Please!"

Mary Anne's anxiety touched her. "I'll be back tomorrow early. And the next day and the day after that. I promise."

Mary Anne gripped Charlotte's hand. She pulled herself up from the pillows and leaned her head against her sister's breast. After a while she spoke. "I don't want to leave Thomas and the children. What will they do without me?" They sat for a few moments with Charlotte holding her sister close, gently stroking her hair.

"I'll be here as long as you need me," Charlotte finally said, "because I love you so very much."

The next day, Charlotte got off to an early start. Kate and Min had settled in well, as she had known they would. Margaret enjoyed her role as grandmother, and there were many new things for the children to see and do. Before setting out in the democrat, Charlotte admonished Kate and Min to behave themselves and Margaret not to spoil them. Knowing her stepmother, she realized this last instruction was the one least likely to be observed.

On the drive into town Charlotte thought about Mary Anne's illness. Dr. Cole had been a family friend as well as physician from the girls' childhoods. Charlotte remembered him noting that Mary Anne was quick to catch seasonal illnesses and that she suffered more and longer from them than anyone else in the family. No one had ever thought much of this. The Whiteheads' elder daughter simply was said to be more delicate than her sister and brothers.

Gradually Mary Anne's illnesses had kept her bedridden more frequently and for longer periods. Her condition was commonly ascribed to her having "weak lungs." Almost four years had passed since Charlotte had pestered Dr. Cole into lending her a general medical textbook from his office library. From reading it late into that same night, she had learned that Mary Anne was suffering from consumption. Over the next while, Charlotte had read Da Costa's *Practice of Medicine* from cover to cover.

"How are you feeling today?"
Mary Anne made a tired face. "About the same."
"Did you have a good night?"

Without waiting for an answer Charlotte felt the wrinkled bed linens. They were damp, as she had thought they would be.

"You must have slept fitfully," she said. She placed the back of her hand against Mary Anne's forehead. "You're still running a fever."

Mary Anne made another face – this time a wry one. "Must you fuss so?"

"Yes, I must."

Charlotte bathed her sister and changed the bed linens. She had barely finished when there was a knock at the door.

"That will be Dr. Cole," Charlotte said. "Thomas told me he was coming by this morning."

As Charlotte went to let him in, Mary Anne drew the bedclothes up to the shirred neck of her nightdress.

"Good morning, Mrs. Ross," Dr. Cole said, his accent as Irish as the River Liffey. "It's always a pleasure to see you back in Clinton." He turned his attention to Mary Anne. "And how is our patient this morning?"

"She's had a feverish night," Charlotte said. "I just finished changing the bed linens."

Dr. Cole sat down by her side. "Still feeling a little warm, are we?"

Mary Anne nodded.

"Have you taken the pills I left you?" He glanced at the prescription bottle on the bedside table, noting it was almost as full as when he had brought it. "Still coughing as much?"

He redirected the question to Charlotte. "Is she?"

"Now and then," Charlotte said.

"Any blood?"

"A little. Not very much."

Dr. Cole gently took down the bedclothes from where Mary Anne had tucked them under her chin. She turned her face away from him, her eyes fixed on a wallpaper daffodil. He undid the top buttons of her nightdress and put his stethoscope to her chest. He listened briefly, then put the instrument back in his coat pocket without comment. There was no change, Charlotte knew. Nor had she expected any. Mary Anne began doing up the buttons of her nightdress, and Dr. Cole turned to Charlotte.

"Has she been eating anything?"

"A little broth."

"That's not enough." He frowned at Mary Anne. "We'll not get our strength back without decent nourishment."

"I don't feel like eating," Mary Anne protested. "Besides, most of the time nothing stays down."

"Well, do your best."

Dr. Cole got up to go. "I'll come by in another day or two."

Charlotte followed him into the hallway, closing the door behind her. "I didn't get here until yesterday," she said. "I've got her taking her medication regularly. I'm trying to interest her in poached eggs, custards and oatmeal gruel."

Dr. Cole nodded his approval. "Will she take liquids?"

"She's been good about that. I've been giving her all the water and tea she can drink, with broths between."

Dr. Cole nodded again. He paused at the top of the stairs. "I

21

take it you intend to spend a lot of time with your sister?"

"As much as needed."

"Good. She needs companionship as much as anything. Someone to help her get her mind off herself. Are her children still here?"

"They're staying with relatives."

"Bring them over whenever she's up to seeing them. I'll be back the day after tomorrow."

"Thank you, doctor."

"No thanks needed. You may be just the tonic your sister needs."

When Charlotte returned to the room, she went to the bottle of pills on the bedside table and shook one out. Then she poured a glass of water from the ironstone jug and handed the pill to Mary Anne. "Here. Take this," she said with mock severity. "Dr. Cole says you must have three each day, and it's time for your second."

Mary Anne frowned at her sister. "Charlotte, I am not a barn swallow."

"I didn't say you were."

They laughed. Mary Anne took the pill from Charlotte and put it in her mouth. Before she could take a drink she started to cough, spilling some of the water over her bedclothes. Charlotte quickly took away the glass. After a few moments, Mary Anne was all right again. After she had sipped a little water, with Charlotte holding the glass to her lips, she smiled apologetically. "I shouldn't laugh and try to drink at the same time."

"It's good to hear you laugh," said Charlotte. "We can always get you dry bedclothes."

Charlotte left soon after this. It was drawing near suppertime. She wanted to be home with Kate and Min at the meal hour, and later to cook up some of the food Dr. Cole had agreed would be good for her sister. When their stepmother asked about Mary Anne, Charlotte repeated what she thought were the most important parts of her conversation with Dr. Cole. Then she asked for Margaret's help, knowing beforehand what her answer would be. It had always been the same, from the September day fifteen years earlier, when she had entered their home and their lives as their stepmother.

"If the children aren't too much for you," Charlotte said, "I'd like to spend most of my days with Mary Anne. I thought I might get there in time to prepare breakfast and not leave until about this time every evening."

"Whatever you think is best."

"You're sure you don't mind? I don't like to give you the responsibility of looking after Kate and Min all day."

"If it were anything but a pleasure I'd say so. I've got help here in the house, and besides, I don't see near enough of them. It will be a treat for all three of us!"

After she had put the children to bed, parrying Kate's persistent questions on when she and Min might visit their aunt Mary Anne, Charlotte went down to the kitchen and started baking bread. It helped take her mind off what she recognized as the advanced state of her sister's illness. Besides, if anything would induce Mary Anne to take solid food, she was confident it was the stone-milled, whole-kernel loaves she would pull from the oven, hot and brown-crusted. Charlotte baked better bread than anyone else in the family.

The next morning she was up at daybreak. She put a wicker basket on the passenger seat of the democrat. In it she had packed loaves of bread and an earthenware crock of baked custard beneath a linen napkin. When she got to the post office, she shooed Mary Anne's husband out of the kitchen and made her sister a nourishing breakfast of poached eggs, tea and toast. Then she made up a tray and carried it to the upstairs bedroom. "Good morning!"

Mary Anne was already awake. She had been listening to the sounds coming from the kitchen. She pouted as Charlotte set the tray on the bedside table. "I did not ask for breakfast."

"I did not ask if you asked," Charlotte replied cheerfully. She leaned over Mary Anne and helped her draw herself up, plumping the pillows. She picked up the pitcher, poured water and took a pill from the bottle. "First this." Charlotte gave the pill to Mary Anne, followed by a sip of water. "Then breakfast."

"I really don't feel like anything."

"I was up half the night baking that bread," Charlotte said, placing the tray before her sister. "Eat."

"Maybe a little toast and tea."

"And some egg."

Mary Anne made a face at Charlotte, but she broke off a corner of toast and dipped it in the yolk of one of the eggs. While

24

her sister picked at her breakfast, Charlotte looked around the room. Two years earlier, when she and David had moved to Montreal and she could no longer help Mary Anne during her illnesses, Thomas had hired a housekeeper to come by once a week. She did the laundry and gave the house a lick and a promise, which Charlotte now decided it was high time someone kept.

Charlotte went down to the kitchen. She filled two pails with hot water from the big copper kettle that sat on the back of the cookstove. Then she put shaved bar soap and a heaping tablespoon of lye into one of the pails. When she went back upstairs with the hot water, two washcloths and a paring knife, Mary Anne had finished her breakfast.

"You did well," Charlotte said, removing the tray.

"I ate as much as I could."

Charlotte hitched up the sleeves of her dress.

"What are you doing?"

"I'm going to give this room a good scrubbing."

"You don't have to do that!"

"It needs it. Besides, you'll feel more comfortable in a clean room."

Over Mary Anne's protests, Charlotte got down on her hands and knees. She soaked one of the cloths in the pail with the soap and lye mixed with hot water and began washing the floor. The other cloth she rinsed and wrung out in clear hot water for mopping up. She used the paring knife to scrape clean where the floor met the baseboards. When she finished, Charlotte sat at her sister's bedside and read aloud from *The Canadian Illustrated News*, which she had brought with her from Montreal. She made a rich chicken broth for Mary Anne's midday meal and a gruel for her supper. She served both with her own good bread and the custard she had brought.

The days and weeks that followed were a repetition of the first. Charlotte rose early to get Kate and Min ready for their grandmother, then drove off to prepare her sister's breakfast. The rest of her day was spent cleaning and cooking, talking with Mary Anne and reading to her, or just sitting by her bedside while she slept until it was time to go home again. Dr. Cole came by once or twice a week.

It was at the end of one of these visits, early in June, that he told Charlotte he wished to speak with her. She followed him from the bedroom, closing the door behind her.

"I want you to know I'm impressed with what you've done for Mary Anne," said Dr. Cole. "I never would have believed the progress she has made over the past while." He looked thoughtfully at Charlotte. "You seem to have an aptitude for caring for the sick."

"The medical textbook you were kind enough to lend me helped," said Charlotte. "Since I moved to Montreal, another doctor has helped me with my studies."

Dr. Cole raised his eyebrows. He had not been aware that Charlotte's interest had lasted over the four years since he had loaned her Da Costa's *Practice of Medicine*.

"Perhaps you know him? Dr. William Hingston?"

Dr. Cole nodded. William Hales Hingston was prominent as a Montreal surgeon and a founding member, two years earlier, of the Canadian Medical Association.

"I know Dr. Hingston only by reputation," said Dr. Cole. "Do you know him well?"

"Quite well. We met while I was summering at my father's house in Glengarry. He is a frequent visitor at a friend's."

"Is Dr. Hingston responsible for your preoccupation with cleanliness in the sickroom? It seems that every time I come to see Mary Anne you are scrubbing down her room, or washing and ironing her bedclothes."

Charlotte laughed. "Come now, Dr. Cole! Surely you don't see me as such a drudge!"

"Heaven forbid," said Dr. Cole, raising his hand in protest. "We are told that cleanliness is next to godliness. Thinking physicians who have read the theories of Louis Pasteur and Joseph Lister are inclined to agree."

"My friend Dr. Hingston certainly does," said Charlotte.

"As do I," said Dr. Cole.

When Charlotte arrived home, she found Margaret busy with her sewing basket in the front room.

"I was beginning to worry," her stepmother said, glancing up as she pulled tight a stitch. "You're later tonight than usual."

"Mary Anne was slow to settle. She had another of her coughing spells."

Margaret clucked her concern.

"Are Kate and Min gone to bed?"

"An hour or so ago."

Margaret looked sharply at Charlotte over her sewing.

"You've got more energy than any two people I know. What with getting away so early and back so late day after day, I should think you'd be concerned about your own well-being."

"I'm just fine," Charlotte reassured her. She knew her step-mother meant well, but she had no time for this discussion. She seized upon Kate and Min as an excuse to go upstairs. "I'll see if the children need tucking in," she said. "Then I think I'll go to bed. You're right, I do feel a little tired."

"Small wonder," Margaret said.

When Charlotte looked in on her two daughters, holding the coal-oil lamp just inside the doorway, she saw that both were asleep. She quietly closed the door again and went to her own room. She set the lamp by some books on a small table by the window. There was no point in waking them, she told herself, just to wish them goodnight. She would see them in the morning and try to get home that evening a little earlier than usual. Charlotte went to the table by the window and sat down. She opened one of the books Dr. Hingston had loaned her before she left Montreal, and hunched down under the yellow glow of the coal-oil lamp. She studied Scanzoni's *Diseases of Women* long into the night.

School closed in Montreal just in time for Charlotte's eldest daughter to celebrate her birthday with her mother and sisters in Clinton. Bella and David arrived by train on the afternoon of Monday, June 28. Charlotte met them at the station with the houseman and the half-covered carriage and pair. When Bella stepped down from the railway car and saw her mother, she ran and threw her arms around her.

"Happy birthday!" Charlotte said laughing, stooping to give her daughter a welcoming kiss and a hug. Then she straightened and embraced her husband, who handed their luggage to George to load onto the rear of the carriage. "Can you stay the weekend?"

David shook his head. "I have to get back tomorrow."

Charlotte made a face, then smiled down at Bella as her daughter tugged at her skirts.

"I'm seven today!"

"I know!" Charlotte said. She took Bella's hand and the three of them walked to the carriage. "We're having a very special dinner tonight with all the things you like to eat and a birthday cake with eight candles on it."

"Eight?" Bella echoed.

"One's for good luck."

They got into the carriage. As George drove them from the station, David asked about Mary Anne.

"She's got some of her strength back," Charlotte told him. "She has good days and bad."

"You said in your last letter that nothing has changed."

"Nothing has, really. I've had long talks with Dr. Cole. The best anyone can do is make her as comfortable as possible. I've been doing that."

David was briefly silent. "How long?" he asked quietly.

"It's hard to say."

They were silent for a while. Driving up Main Street between the neat rows of Clinton shops prompted Charlotte to ask David how things were at Whitehead and Ross.

"Well enough. Sometimes it bothers me, though. More and more people are moving west. Half the people in Montreal, if you can believe all you hear."

"You've thought of going?"

"At times. There's real opportunity, I should think, if you're among the early ones."

Charlotte smiled at her husband. "You sound serious."

David shrugged.

They fell silent again. David had never mentioned this before. Charlotte wondered what life would be like in what was called Rupert's Land and the North-West. Primitive, she decided. Probably very hard, but challenging. And where there was challenge, there were rewards. She would not mind going west with her husband and family. She would welcome any new turn their lives took, God willing, and all it had to offer.

When they got to the house there was a noisy reunion between Bella and her sisters, contrasting with David and Margaret's quiet pleasure at their first meeting since Christmas. Whether it was their common Scots ancestry, or David's respect for Margaret's devotion to Charlotte and her three other stepchildren, they shared a close relationship. While the children played outside, Charlotte and David took tea with Margaret in the parlour. When Charlotte finished, she went upstairs to unpack David's bag. She was at the bureau, putting away some of David's things, when he entered. Charlotte turned. He was standing by the table near the window. He picked up one of the textbooks on the table and leafed through it.

"These are new," he said.

"Dr. Hingston loaned them to me before I left Montreal. He thought I might put them to good use while I was here."

David gave her a knowing look. "I'm sure you are."

Charlotte watched him put down the book and wondered if she were this transparent to her husband. She had borrowed the first book from Dr. Cole just to learn more about her sister's illness. Since then she had become involved in the study of medicine generally, reading everything she could find on symptoms, diagnoses and treatments. In this she had been encouraged and helped by Dr. Hingston. Standing now in front of David she felt a sense of self-betrayal, as though she had left some window on her inner self unshuttered.

Later she realized that David must have seen this in her eyes. He suddenly laughed outright, seizing her around the waist and pulling her down beside him on the bed. She gave a small cry of surprise and he put his finger to her lips, inclining his head towards the doorway that led downstairs. They were silent for a moment, looking into each other's eyes.

"I've missed you," David finally whispered.

"I'm glad," Charlotte replied with a smile. "I'd hate to be the only one."

David kissed her. Close in his embrace, she knew that tonight she would not be burning the midnight oil.

Charlotte's father had wanted to be home for his granddaughter's birthday. Although the House had recessed for the summer the previous week, Joseph had had to remain in Ottawa on business.

"He plans to be home within the next few days," Margaret said as they sat down to dinner. "I certainly hope he is. He has to return to Ottawa at the end of July for the fall sessions. I scarcely see your father any more, now that he's in federal politics."

When dinner was over, Bella opened her gifts. David had brought from Montreal a china doll exquisite in bonneted ringlets, a full skirt with petticoats, and high-button shoes. The rest of the family gave her everything she needed, from miniature linens and china to a table and four chairs, to hold a children's tea party. Charlotte and David left Bella pouring for her doll and two sisters. Margaret watched over the children while their parents went to see Mary Anne.

Throughout the visit, David was ill at ease. It was obvious how serious his sister-in-law's condition was. David had been born in Ferintosh, Scotland, in the long shadow of the clan castle. He had been brought up God-fearing, loyal to clan and family, law-abiding, hard-working and as close with his mouth as he was with his purse. Charlotte knew her husband was not a man to squander anything, including sentiment, and she respected this. After a decent interval, he excused himself and went downstairs to talk with Thomas. He was relieved when it came time to go home.

"Mary Anne was pleased by your visit," Charlotte said.

David untied the reins from the hitching post in front of the post office. As he stepped up to the driver's seat beside his wife, he tugged at a corner of his squared beard. Charlotte gave him a sideways look. Her husband was a good-looking man, eyes set well between high cheekbones, his brow broadened by a receding hairline. Although he was ten years older than she was, in some ways he seemed younger and was less sure of himself. She placed a hand over the one that held the reins.

"You were just fine," she said.

David got up early the next morning and caught the train at 6:25 for Stratford. There was a later service, but this was an express that gave him his best connections to Toronto and Montreal. After driving her husband to the station, Charlotte returned to her daily routine of caring for Mary Anne.

Charlotte had been looking forward to seeing her father just as much as Margaret was. When his telegram arrived a few days later declaring that he was leaving Ottawa and would be in Clinton the day following, she took part in the preparations for his arrival that began that same evening. Charlotte baked bread. Margaret had the houseman polish harnesses in the barn and bring to a high shine the half-covered carriage and the democrat. In the morning, his wife was soon bustling back and forth between the summer kitchen and the cellar cold room. Margaret planned the dinner menu and was preparing the main dishes herself: carrot soup, roast beef with Yorkshire pudding, and baked apple in custard sauce.

All went well until mid-afternoon, when Mary Anne took one of her abrupt turns for the worse. While Charlotte held her and massaged her back, she coughed herself limp, spitting blood and phlegm from her congested lungs. Charlotte was unable to go with the houseman to meet her father's train. When George called for her at the post office she told him she was unable to leave Mary Anne, but to advise Mr. Whitehead that she would join him at dinner. This, too, turned out to be impossible. By the time she had made her sister comfortable for the night, it was well past the dinner hour. When she finally got home, the children had been put to bed and her father was waiting for her in the parlour. Margaret was in the summer kitchen making a fresh pot of tea. Charlotte walked to her father and embraced him.

"I'm sorry, Father. I couldn't get away any sooner."

"I understand. Margaret has been telling me how devoted you have been to your sister. How is she?"

"She was resting when I left. She's had a trying day. One of the worst she's had in some time."

"Her condition? Is it just as critical?"

"The same."

Her father scowled. Joseph was fifty-five. He was heavy-set, with a black spade beard going silver. His manner was brusquely confident. Charlotte realized that Mary Anne's illness was both an insult and an enigma to her father. He not only felt personally wronged, but powerless to do anything about it.

"I suppose it's too late to visit her now?"

"It would be better in the morning."

"I would have come straight from the station, but I decided it was best to wait until we spoke."

"It was. You wouldn't have wanted to see her – not the way she was today."

Joseph nodded.

Charlotte thought to change the subject. "How are things in Ottawa?"

Her father looked relieved. "Good for the future of this country. The Hudson's Bay Company is giving up control of Rupert's Land and the North-West. They'll soon be part of the Dominion."

Margaret interrupted with the tea tray. The conversation changed to family matters.

"Have you seen Charles and the children?" Joseph asked his daughter.

"Soon after I arrived," said Charlotte. "Hanna came by to visit with Mary Anne. She brought the children with her."

Hanna was five years older than Charlotte. Her parents were United Empire Loyalists who had crossed the border into what was now Ontario, and had settled in Smiths Falls. Charles and Hanna had a six-year-old daughter and two younger sons. Margaret McDonald was named for Charles's stepmother and their first-born son, Joseph, for his father. Their second son was Charles Jr.

They talked a while longer, deciding on the next morning for Joseph's visit with Mary Anne. Finally Charlotte wished her father and Margaret good night and went upstairs. After she had looked in on the children and changed into her nightdress, she took a book from her bureau drawer and sat with it at the table. It was a textbook that she chose to keep hidden from anyone who happened into her bedroom. She knew it would have shocked the Victorian gentlemen in her family and possibly even Margaret as well. The thought made her smile a little. She moved the lamp closer and turned to where she had left off in Gray's *Anatomy*, with its physically explicit studies of men and women.

The next day Charlotte breakfasted with the children and was gone before her father had awakened. It was not until mid-morning that he arrived to visit with his ailing daughter. Mary Anne was feeling much better. The three of them had a pleasant time. Even so, Charlotte knew how difficult it was for their father to sit and carry on a cheerful conversation, as though his elder daughter was just briefly indisposed and would soon be well again. Serious illness was wretchedly difficult, Charlotte had learned over the past while, both for those who were ill and those who loved and provided care for them.

Finally, Joseph awkwardly tugged his gold pocket watch from his waistcoat, snapped open the cover, and frowned at its Roman face.

"Well, I must be going now, Mary Anne." His voice was gruff. "You get well soon."

Charlotte hung back when their father abruptly turned and left the room. When she joined him a few moments later at the top of the stairs, he had regained control of himself.

"I appreciate what you're doing for Mary Anne," he said. "We all do."

For the month the House remained in summer recess, Charlotte had no concerns about how to keep Bella, Kate and Min occupied. Joseph was the doting grandfather. Scarcely a day passed that he didn't find some excuse to drive about Clinton in his half-covered carriage and pair, proudly showing off his three granddaughters. In some ways, too, it was a good time for Charlotte. The long days of mid-summer gave her late evening light to work in the garden, which she enjoyed. The white rose bushes her mother had brought from England, which Charlotte had transplanted from their original homestead near The Corners, had never bloomed so beautifully. She loved her mother's roses. They brought back patchwork memories of her English childhood. She kept a fresh bouquet on the table by Mary Anne's bed, regularly replacing it before the room lost its sweet fragrance.

Early in August, shortly after her father returned to Ottawa, Charlotte acted on Margaret Hale's invitation to visit. The post office was a clearing house for news of anything of interest that happened in Clinton. Charlotte had heard from Thomas that Sarah Hale, Margaret's mother-in-law, had arrived from Philadelphia to spend some time with her son and his family.

Charlotte had never met Sarah Hale, but she was interested

in many of the ideas expressed in *Godey's Lady's Book*, the magazine she edited. The first woman editor of a major American magazine, she was a controversial figure. While she held the sanctity of the family as inviolate, she believed in the right of women, single or married, to a career. Her support had helped create Vassar College for Women in Poughkeepsie, New York. At the same time, she opposed giving women the vote on the grounds that they were above anything as base as politics. By feminists she was thought to be an eccentric; by traditionalists, a radical.

Charlotte drove to the Hales' house directly from her day with her sister. She was shown into the parlour by the housegirl, and given tea with Margaret and her husband. They enquired after Mary Anne, expressing regret at the seriousness of her condition. The conversation turned to Horatio's success, along with the Reverend A.K. McDonald, in getting a new secondary school for the town. They had finally managed to get the Department of Education, in Toronto, to accept two girls as the equivalent of one boy. This gave Clinton the enrolment it needed to qualify for a building grant.

"We were ten boys short," said Horatio. "Until now, girls didn't count."

On this remark, his mother entered the room. Charlotte had been told she was eighty years old and always wore mourning black. As Charlotte stood, she thought she understood at last the meaning of the word *matriarch*.

"Sit down," Sarah Hale commanded, waiting for the order to

be carried out before taking the chair opposite.

"This is Mrs. David Ross – Charlotte," said Margaret. "I've spoken to you about her and her sister, Mary Anne."

Her mother-in-law nodded, shrewdly but not unkindly appraising their young visitor.

"I enjoy your magazine," Charlotte said.

"Thank you. I don't think it's as good today as it was thirty or so years ago, when some of our finest authors wrote for us. Nevertheless, *Godey's* is still the acknowledged authority on America's manners and mores."

"This is one of the reasons I came to visit," said Charlotte. "I would like your opinion on the idea of a wife and mother studying to become a female doctor."

The older woman gave Charlotte a stern look. "I have no opinion about female anything," she said finally. "Cows, sows and hens are female. We are none of these, nor are we chattels of men, but women!"

Charlotte was momentarily taken aback. "A woman doctor, then," she said, recovering, emphasizing the word *woman*.

"Why not? Do you have the talent for it? I assume it's you we're talking about."

"I have been caring for my chronically ill sister and studying medical books," Charlotte said. "A friend who is a physician and surgeon has given me a great deal of encouragement."

"Then do it, girl! America's first woman doctor graduated nineteen years ago. If Elizabeth Blackwell can do it, so can you." She raised a cautioning hand. "Mind you, a woman's first duty is to her family. I had five children of my own and I believe that every wife and mother should be an inspiration to her husband and family. I also believe that there's a role for women in the professions. If she has a mind to, an intelligent woman can do both."

Charlotte required no more convincing. A while later, as she drove off from the Hales' in her father's democrat, she recognized that her meeting with Sarah Hale had simply set her feet more surely on a path she had already chosen. Charlotte considered Sarah Hale a remarkable woman. Not only had she worked with famous writers like Edgar Allan Poe, but she was a famous writer herself. A rhyme from one of her books, *Poems for Our Children*, already was one of the most popular ever written.

Kate and Min were asleep when Charlotte got home, but Bella lay awake. Charlotte entered their room, shielding the lamp with one hand so she would not disturb the two sleeping children.

"Mother?"

"Shhhh!" Charlotte whispered to Bella. "You'll wake your sisters."

She walked softly to her eldest daughter's bedside and sat down.

"Do you remember 'Mary's Lamb'? We learned it together when you were very young."

Bella nodded. "'Mary had a little lamb,'" she quoted softly, "'whose fleece was white as snow. . . .'"

"'And everywhere that Mary went,'" Charlotte finished,

touching Bella's nose with her fingertip, "'the lamb was sure to go!'"

Bella giggled at this unexpected game her mother was playing. "That rhyme was written many years ago," Charlotte said, "by a young woman visiting a place called Wales who saw a little girl tending sheep in a meadow. The woman was Sarah Hale, and I have just come from having tea with her."

Mary Anne's condition worsened over the next two weeks. She slept for longer periods both day and night, coming fitfully awake and calling out for her sister. Charlotte found herself having to arrive earlier and leave later. She had little time now for the children and she was doubly grateful to Margaret for her willingness to act as a mother to them. More often than not, Charlotte left the house before it was fully light and did not return until some time after dark. She frequently went for prescriptions to Watts and Co., or had William deliver them, which gave rise to a shared joke – that they saw more of each other than any others in the family. Dr. Cole looked in on Mary Anne every other day. As he had told Charlotte in April, there was little he could do for her sister that hadn't already been done. All that remained was seeing to her personal comfort, which Charlotte was capable of doing better than anyone else.

It was near the end of the summer, after one of his regular visits, that Charlotte got into a thought-provoking discussion with Dr. Cole on women and medicine.

"I might have been able to help Mary Anne," he said, "if she had come to me sooner. Lord knows how many women's lives are lost to Victorian modesty." His expression darkened. "Every physician has women patients who wait too long to be examined, then insist it be done under bedsheets!"

"Perhaps the need is for women doctors," said Charlotte.

Dr. Cole looked at her thoughtfully. "I wouldn't go so far as that," he said finally. "None of our medical schools accepts women. Other considerations aside, that's the biggest obstacle.

"There are three that do in the United States."

"It makes no difference. No foreign graduate can practise here without completing prescribed sessions of study domestically."

"None of which are open to women."

"Exactly. In time this may change. What's needed now is a more sensible attitude by women towards their physicians."

"That's difficult for some," said Charlotte. "It's a matter of strict moral upbringing, even religious belief."

Dr. Cole shook his head, turning to go. He hesitated. "Mrs. Ross."

"Yes?"

"Are you contemplating studying to be a physician?"

"I have given it some thought."

"Have you considered nursing? It is less demanding and would seem more suited to women."

Charlotte bridled. "I have discovered that nursing demands great dedication and special skills; the patience of Job, as well. But if I am to do medical work, it will be as a doctor."

"I see." Dr. Cole studied the slight young woman who spoke so defiantly. "I am not in favour of female doctors," he said finally. "On the other hand, I feel you might make a good one."

Before Charlotte could recover from her surprise at this unexpected remark, Dr. Cole turned and was gone.

In the early morning darkness of the first Friday in September, Charlotte was awakened by a loud commotion at the front door of the house. She quickly got up and put on her night robe and slippers. She lit the lamp by her bed and hurried with it into the hallway. She heard Bella call out to her, and then Kate and Min. As she passed Margaret's room, her stepmother opened the door. She was holding a lighted lamp in one hand and clutching her nightdress to her throat with the other.

"What in the name of heaven?"

"It sounds like Thomas," said Charlotte. She walked quickly to the top of the stairs. She was halfway down to the entry hall when she looked back and saw her stepmother standing motionless at the door to her room. "The children, Margaret! They're frightened!"

Margaret abruptly became aware of the cries coming from down the hallway. When Bella stumbled sleepily from her room, she was there to hush and put her arms around her.

Charlotte unbolted and opened the door to her brother-in-law.

"It's Mary Anne. She's taken a bad turn – the worst yet."

"I'll get dressed."

Thomas shook his head. "There's no time."

Charlotte put down her lamp on the entry-hall table and pulled her night robe closer. Margaret came downstairs and walked quickly to where Charlotte and Thomas stood at the front door.

"Mary Anne needs me," said Charlotte. "I'm going with Thomas." They climbed into the buggy he had tethered at the front of the house.

"Tell the children I'll be back soon!" Charlotte called out.

Thomas slapped the reins smartly across the horse's back. From the doorway, Margaret watched the swaying light of the buggy's lantern until it was lost in the darkness.

Thomas reined up in front of the post office. Charlotte jumped down and ran directly into the house. She found Mary Anne lying quite still, her eyes vacantly open. Charlotte took hold of her wrist and felt for her pulse. Then she picked up the small looking glass that lay beside the ironstone jug and wash-bowl, and held it to her sister's lips. She kept it there longer than was needed, knowing that it would not mist over. Finally, when she heard her brother-in-law's footsteps on the stairs, Charlotte laid the looking glass back down on the table. She gently closed her sister's eyes and sat down beside her. She waited for Thomas with her hands clasped tightly in her lap.

CHAPTER THREE

Clinton, Fall, 1869

*T*HE SKY WEPT SOFTLY on the morning they buried
Mary Anne. What David called a Scotch mist began to
fall as the lengthy cortège left Clinton's white clapboard
Presbyterian church. Those mourners with convertible carriages had their carriage tops raised. The rest sat hunched under
umbrellas or stoically erect in damp suits and bonneted dresses.
Thomas and the two children rode in a covered carriage immediately behind the hearse. This was fully enclosed with the
ornaments of death carved in black relief, the coffin concealed
behind curtained windows. It was drawn by two plumed black
horses in black bridles and harnesses.

The Whiteheads' half-covered carriage was driven by the
houseman. Margaret, Charlotte and Hanna sat opposite Joseph,
David and Charles. William rode with the Ross and Whitehead
children in the third carriage. Thomas's brother and two sisters
came next, followed by a long line of carriages and buggies
bearing more distant relatives and friends.

At the graveside, Joseph and Charles stood by Mary Anne's
husband. David held an umbrella for Charlotte. She stood hand
in hand with her sister's two children. Josie and William looked

straight ahead, both too young to fully understand, but caught up in the melancholy. Each held a small nosegay of white roses Charlotte had given them.

The Reverend McDonald delivered a brief eulogy of the deceased as a devoted wife and mother. He stooped and picked up a handful of dirt. "For as much as it has pleased Almighty God to take unto Himself the life of our sister here dedicated, we therefore commit her body to the ground." He sprinkled dirt on the coffin. "Earth to earth, ashes to ashes, dust to dust, in the sure and certain hope of the resurrection of the dead through our Lord Jesus Christ."

Charlotte gently urged Josie and William forward. The two children walked to the graveside and laid the nosegays on their mother's coffin. Their father joined them, taking each by the hand. They stood there together as the plain pine box was lowered by its rope sling into the ground.

Charlotte was lost in reminiscence. She gave a start when David lightly touched her elbow. When he motioned towards the waiting carriage, she slowly turned away from her sister's graveside. She could not do the same from her memories.

Charlotte was sixteen years old when she became a boarder at the Convent of the Sacred Heart at Sault-au-Récollet, on the Island of Montreal. It was the first time she and Mary Anne were separated since the death of their mother eight years earlier.

Charlotte was preparing to leave during the last week in

April. Her sister was helping her pack. "I will miss you," said Mary Anne.

"And I you."

"It seems so long a time we'll be apart."

Charlotte paused in the act of folding a dress. "Only fourteen months," she said. "From next week until Father comes for me the second week in July."

Mary Anne took the dress from Charlotte. She busied herself unnecessarily with refolding it. "Well, no doubt the time will fly. I'll have your share of the house and farm chores, and someone has to help Margaret keep an eye on William."

Charlotte's eyes widened, and she cried out in mock protest. "You make me feel guilty I'm going!"

Mary Anne laughed as she carefully placed the dress in the trunk. "Don't be silly! You know I'd just as soon stay here as be packed off to a convent. Besides," she added matter-of-factly, "you've always been the bright one. Everyone knows that."

Charlotte and her cousin Emma, one of Senator McDonald's daughters, enjoyed their time at the convent. Even so, Charlotte missed Mary Anne and sometimes felt guilty; not because she had left her sister to do her share of the household work, as they had joked, but because she alone had been given this opportunity to improve herself. As well as scholastics, the nuns excelled in teaching the drawingroom arts. During her fourteen months at Sault-au-Récollet, Charlotte studied voice and piano. She became skilled at embroidery and needlework. On the *jour du prix*, when prizes were given for excellence on the day the students left for home, Charlotte was awarded the medal in French.

She had all this and more to tell Mary Anne when she got back to Clinton in mid-July. She ran from the carriage into the house. She was brought up short by her stepmother, standing at the foot of the stairs with a finger to her lips.

"Go quietly," Margaret cautioned. "Your sister is having one of her poorly spells."

Charlotte's husband and father left by train together the day after the funeral. Joseph made connections at Prescott with the St. Lawrence and Ottawa Railway. David stayed on through to Montreal. Charlotte remained behind to help Thomas and the children over their first few difficult days without Mary Anne.

"We'll be all right," Thomas assured her.

Charlotte had brought clean laundry and baking with her. She stayed to cook supper. Back home that evening, she put her own three children to bed early. She had decided to discuss her plans with her stepmother. When Charlotte came downstairs from the children's bedroom, Margaret was reading the newspaper by lamplight. She lowered the pages of *The New Era* and smiled at her stepdaughter.

"Are the children asleep already?"

"Almost before I kissed them good night."

"They've had a busy day, helping George down at the stable."

"He's good to them."

"He likes children," Margaret said, returning to her newspaper.

"There's something I'd like to talk with you about."

Charlotte's stepmother looked at her enquiringly. She folded the newspaper in her lap.

"I intend to apply for entrance to medical school."

Margaret nodded. "That doesn't surprise me."

"It doesn't?"

"I couldn't help but notice the medical books in your bedroom. Some nights I have trouble sleeping. When I came downstairs to warm some milk I would see the light under your door. It was always very late."

"Well, what do you think?"

Margaret didn't reply at once. When she did, it was cautiously. "I think everyone should do what they feel is right for them. Providing, of course, no one else is wronged because of it."

"You mean David and the children," Charlotte said. "Whatever I do, they will always come first."

"Could you be sure, Charlotte? I would think medical studies are very demanding, and carrying on a practice even more so."

"I believe if you want to do something badly enough you can adjust to anything."

"I suppose that's true," Margaret mused. "It's quite unusual for a woman to become a physician, but not unheard of. I'm told some missionaries have, before going off to some strange place or other with their husbands."

"I intend to practise here at home. There is a great need for women doctors."

"Where would you take your studies?"

"Probably in Philadelphia."

"There's nowhere closer? Montreal, or perhaps Toronto?"

"Nowhere that will accept women. There are three that do in the United States. One is the Woman's Medical College of Pennsylvania."

"Well, at least you have relatives in Philadelphia. You must remember my speaking of Aunt Annie and Aunt Johan?"

Charlotte nodded. Both were on the McDonald side of the family.

"You haven't mentioned this to anyone else?" said Margaret. "Not even David?"

Charlotte thought back to the day two months before, when her husband had brought Bella to Clinton, and how transparent she felt when he had remarked on the medical books at her bedside.

"I haven't told David yet," she said, "but I don't think he'll be surprised."

"David may not be," Margaret acknowledged. "But I'm sure your father simply won't hear of it."

"That's why I wanted to speak with you."

"To enlist an ally?" Margaret smiled. "Quite frankly, Charlotte, it's not something I would do myself. I'm not even sure I approve. My own life is my family and my home. Like most women, I don't need or even want anything more." She smiled again, this time resignedly. "But then, I suppose the world would be a dreary place if everyone thought and did the same. I promise I'll give you all the help I can."

Charlotte reached and placed a hand over her stepmother's. "Don't doubt for one moment," Margaret said, "that you are going to need it."

CHAPTER FOUR

Montreal, Fall, 1869

CHARLOTTE AND THE CHILDREN returned to Montreal a week or so after the funeral. Bella missed the opening of school by two weeks, but she had a quick mind, and her mother did not doubt that she would catch up. David was pleased to have the family together again, and Charlotte was glad to be home. The children, too, were happy to be back, although they declared they missed their grandmother, the farm animals, and the houseman and his wife, in that order.

Mary Anne's final illness had been a strain on everyone, but especially on Charlotte. She knew it was not the nearly five months of physical care she had given her sister. She prided herself on having strength and endurance well beyond that suggested by her slight body. Nor was it the emotional involvement. No, instead it was the agony of knowing that, whatever she did for Mary Anne, it was not enough to keep her from dying. That had been the worst of it.

On the morning after their return from Clinton, Charlotte took Bella to school. Then she drove to Upper St. Urbain in Montreal. Dr. Hingston had apprenticed as a pharmacist while studying medicine at McGill University. A year's postgraduate study at hospitals in London, Edinburgh and Dublin had qualified him as a licentiate with the Royal College of Physicians and Surgeons. Returning to Montreal, he had soon established the reputation that had led to his appointment as chief surgeon at Hôtel Dieu Hospital.

Dr. Hingston studied the young woman who sat across the office desk from him. "So you have made up your mind to apply to an American medical school?"

"Yes."

He had been impressed with Charlotte Ross from the moment they had been introduced by mutual friends two summers ago in Glengarry. Out of their infrequent meetings since, socially or when Charlotte visited him at Hôtel Dieu to borrow from his medical library, had arisen a special relationship. Neither the forty-year-old surgeon, nor the woman he looked upon as an interesting, perhaps even promising protégée, had ever chosen to examine it closely. "Have you decided which college?"

"I think the one in Philadelphia. I have a maiden aunt I could stay with, two aunts, actually. I also have a friend, Sarah Hale."

"The editor of the magazine?"

Charlotte nodded. "I know her son Horatio and his wife from Clinton. I met Mrs. Hale while she was visiting with them last month. She's a remarkable woman."

Dr. Hingston got up and walked to the front of his desk. "Well, with relatives and friends you'd be better off in Philadelphia. It may be difficult enough to get David's approval. Your going off alone to a strange city will not impress him; nor your father, either."

Charlotte already had given this much thought. She expected she could answer whatever reservations her husband might have. Convincing her father, she knew, would be more difficult. She had decided these were problems she would deal with when the time came.

"How is David, by the way?"

"He's fine," Charlotte said. "He was saddened by my sister's death, as everyone who knew her was."

"It must have been difficult for you."

"It was for all of us."

Dr. Hingston returned to his desk and sat down. He dipped his pen in the inkwell and scribbled a note to himself. "I will make enquiries of the Woman's Medical College of Pennsylvania."

Charlotte rose to go. "You are a wonderful help to me," she said. "I'm still studying the books you loaned me before I left for Clinton."

Dr. Hingston quickly got to his feet and walked her to the door. "Keep them as long as you wish," he said.

"You're sure you don't mind making enquiries for me? I feel it is an imposition."

Dr. Hingston stood with his hand on the doorknob. "My dear Mrs. Ross, whatever I might do for you would never be anything less than a pleasure."

He opened the door and Charlotte walked out into the

corridor. When she reached the far end of the hall she knew he was still watching after her. She looked back and waved to him.

Early in October, when the maples on Mount Royal were turning flamboyant, and the days were getting shorter and sharper, Charlotte received the letter she was expecting from Hôtel Dieu. She dropped the rest of the mail on the entry-hall table and hurried up to her room. She tore open the envelope while she crossed the floor and seated herself at the small escritoire by the window. Inside were a letter of reference and a covering note.

Hôtel Dieu Hospital, Oct. 5

Dear Mrs. Ross:
You will find enclosed my testimonial to your qualifications, both personal and practical, towards entering the study of medicine. Birth and school records and two other references are required.

Address your application to Mrs. E.H. Cleveland, M.D., Secretary of the Faculty, Woman's Medical College of Pennsylvania, 1800 Mount Vernon Street, Philadelphia.

Please keep me advised of your progress and be assured that if I can be of further assistance, I am, your obedient servant,

William Hales Hingston, M.D., L.R.C.S.

Charlotte got up and walked to the bureau. She rummaged through the top drawer and withdrew an envelope containing her baptismal certificate and school graduation diploma. She put these on the writing desk with Dr. Hingston's letter. Then she sat down and began her letter to Dr. Cleveland. She decided

56

to give the Reverend McDonald, and Sister Trincano, of the Convent of the Sacred Heart, as references. Over the period of her residence there, she and the mother superior had become good friends.

Later that day, when David arrived home from the store, he found Charlotte humming about the kitchen waiting supper for him. The children had already eaten and were outside playing, taking advantage of the last while of waning daylight.

"You're in good spirits," said David.

Charlotte smiled over the dinner she set before him. "Does it show that much? I'm happy, that's all."

David helped himself to a slice of bread. "Any special reason?"

"No," Charlotte said. "Just being alive and everyone well."

"You're still remembering Mary Anne." It was a statement, more than a question.

"I wasn't, right then."

Charlotte frowned, correcting herself. "Maybe in a way I was. When you care for someone who is so ill for so long a time, it's not something you soon forget."

"You did the best you could for her."

"Yes. Then."

The qualification was lost on David. Charlotte watched him concentrate on his dinner. She reassured herself that she was not being deceptive. All that afternoon, after she had posted her letter to Philadelphia, Charlotte had been nagged by doubts over whether she should tell David. She finally decided that she was not obliged to reveal her plans to anyone; not until, and if, she were accepted. That would be time enough, she assured herself, to bring everything out in the open – first with her husband, then with her father. Still, as she sat watching David, she felt a little uneasy. This was just the second decision of any real consequence she had ever made on her own. The first had been to marry and make the dutiful transition from being Joseph Whitehead's loving and obedient daughter to being David Ross's loving and obedient wife.

The same week in mid-May that Rupert's Land was renamed Manitoba before becoming the fifth province, Charlotte received her reply from Philadelphia. After such a long wait, she tore open the envelope in the entry hall. Inside was a congratulatory note of acceptance from Dr. Emeline Cleveland. She had also sent along a copy of the *Twenty-First Annual Announcement*, setting out courses, fees, neighbourhood boarding facilities and the Eighteenth Annual Commencement list.

"The degree of doctor of medicine," Charlotte read aloud, "was conferred by the President, T. Morris Perot, Esq., upon the following named ladies."

She paused before silently studying the list of that year's handful of graduates, all from the eastern United States. The names meant nothing to Charlotte, but she read them with as much interest as though they were family. In a way, she told herself, they are. In just three years she would be one of those ladies. The degree of doctor of medicine would be conferred on her, too, by Mr. Perot. The thought brought a mounting sense of excitement that carried her lightly up the stairs to her room. She sat down on the edge of the bed and began reading through the Commencement notice. It did not occur to her to question whether she was able to become one of these few women. She had made up her mind that with determination, hard work and God's help it was something she would do.

It was almost ten o'clock that evening when Charlotte closed her sewing box. She had been trying without much success to concentrate on her needlepoint while David read *The Montreal Witness*.

"All through for the night?" he asked as she got to her feet.

"Yes. My eyes are tired. I thought I'd get an early to bed."

The clock on the mantel board chimed the hour, reminding David that it needed winding. He rose, folding his newspaper in the seat behind him. "I'll be up shortly," he said.

Charlotte picked up the lamp by her chair and walked from the parlour. When David joined her upstairs she was seated in her nightdress at the dressing table. Charlotte knew he enjoyed watching her. She silently counted off the hundred strokes she gave her hair each night before she went to bed.

"I saw to the children," Charlotte said. "Kate was out from under the bedclothes again. She's so restless!"

"I've noticed."

"I tucked her in."

Charlotte had reached 100. With one more for good measure, she laid her silver hairbrush on the dressing table. She stayed seated, turning to face her husband. "I had a letter today."

"From Joseph?" David pulled his nightshirt down over his head and began doing up the buttons. "What did he have to say?"

"It wasn't from Father."

David sat on the edge of the bed.

"It was from the Woman's Medical College of Pennsylvania."

David remained silent.

"They've accepted my application for entrance this fall."

Charlotte had not been certain how her husband would react. She was not prepared for his unchanged expression.

"I'm happy for you," he said.

"You're not surprised?"

"Only that you waited until now to tell me. Otherwise, no. I remember last summer we made some little joke about it. I knew then that you'd been wanting to enter medicine for some time."

"For going on five years now," Charlotte admitted. "Ever since Mary Anne became seriously ill."

"And you began reading medical books."

Charlotte nodded. "At first it was just an idea. It never occurred to me that it could ever come to anything. Then I got involved in the books Dr. Hingston loaned me. He has been very encouraging. So have some others."

"Who?"

"Sarah Hale, when she was visiting in Clinton last summer. And Dr. Cole" – Charlotte made a small frown that quickly became a smile – "although he doesn't approve of women doctors. And Margaret, who doesn't actually approve either, but has promised her support, dear soul! And of course, Dr. Hingston."

David now did show surprise. "They all knew before I did?"

Charlotte got up and went to her husband. She took his hand and sat by his side. "I didn't think to bother you with it. Not until I was sure I'd been accepted. You've been working long hours these past months. I thought you had enough on your mind without this."

"Well," David said, "I can't argue with that. Does Joseph know?"

"No. In the family just Margaret, and now you."

"You'll have to spend much of your time at school. Where?"

"Philadelphia."

"For how long?"

"Three years, from October to March."

David considered this. "Half of each year."

"Less than that. Twenty weeks, actually."

For the first time he looked doubtful. "It's a long absence and a distant city. Are you sure you've given this enough thought?"

"There's no place closer," Charlotte said quickly. "It won't be much change for you and the children, living here with your family. Bella's in school all day. Kate and Min aren't any trouble."

Lately, David had been travelling for Whitehead and Ross as much as three and four weeks at a time. The children were fond of their paternal grandparents and the Rosses' housegirl. If necessary, it would be no great problem to bring in someone just to look after them.

"Where would you stay?"

"With Aunt Annie and Aunt Johan," said Charlotte. "It's not as though I have no family or friends in Philadelphia. There's Sarah Hale, too."

"You have thought it through, haven't you."

"Yes."

"Where would you practise?"

"Here in Montreal."

"Would the authorities let you?"

"I'll know that when the time comes. Things have to change. There has to be a choice for women who prefer a woman doctor."

David nodded. "I agree."

Charlotte got up and brought the lamp to her bedside table. When David had gotten under the bedclothes, she cupped her hand at the chimney and blew out the light.

"You'd best write Joseph this week," said David. "He'll need time to get used to the idea."

"I'd planned to do that tomorrow."

"We'll have to speak to my family. I don't imagine there will be any problem, at least not with your being away. They may not approve of your becoming a doctor."

"It won't matter to me," Charlotte said. "Will it to you?"

"No."

They fell silent. After a while Charlotte guessed David had fallen off to sleep. She lay awake thinking how like him it was to let her have her head. So many husbands wouldn't have. She wondered if she would have done it anyway, with or without his permission.

"Charlotte?" David's voice came unexpectedly, and she turned to face him.

"Yes?"

"You know I'll give you all the help I can." He paused. "You'll do well. I know you will."

Charlotte reached out her hand for his. She wanted him to know how grateful she was for his understanding and how glad she was she had married him. When she felt his hand close over hers and urge her to him, her smile came tender in the darkness.

The next morning, as David had predicted, no problems arose from their announcement to his family. At first his parents were unbelieving that their daughter-in-law, at twenty-seven, intended to abandon her family for almost six months of the year to return to school in a strange city. The fact that their son not only accepted, but also approved of, his wife's decision eliminated whatever reservations they might have had. David's parents were typical Scots in their regard for scholarship. They had overruling respect for anyone with the mind and discipline to study medicine, and said so. Privately, after David had gone to work and Charlotte was seeing to the children, they shook their heads over the fact that this doctor not only would be a woman, but also would be their own daughter-in-law.

As David's parents had been agreeable, Charlotte knew that her own father would be difficult. For some time after the houseman had driven Bella to school, she sat at the escritoire composing a letter to Joseph. Finally it was finished. She read it over twice, looking for ways that might make the letter more plausible to his eyes and more persuasive to hers. It was no use. She knew that, no matter how she worded it, her father would look upon her decision to study medicine as unacceptable. She compressed her lips. She was a grown woman. She had her husband's approval. Her father would simply have to realize he had no say in the matter. On this thought she folded the letter into its envelope. She took some consolation from David's parting remark that at least it would break the ground before she met with her father in six weeks' time at Glengarry.

CHAPTER ❦ FIVE

Glengarry, Summer, 1870

*B*ECAUSE THEY SO ENJOYED GLENGARRY, Charlotte and her family chose to miss the parades and day-long celebrations in Montreal that in three years had become tradition on July 1 – Dominion Day. That morning they boarded the train that ran between Montreal and Toronto at half past eight. Less than two hours later they were met by carriage at Lancaster, Glengarry County, on the Ontario side of the St. Lawrence River.

As the carriage that Margaret had sent for them rolled along the shoreline road, Charlotte shared in the children's excitement. Through gaps in the trees she pointed out the distant swing of white sails as a square-rigged St. Lawrence trader changed tack off Quebec's south shore. They laughed as it staggered upwind like a drunken sailor, its sails flapping and filling from starboard to port.

The carriage also staggered as it turned onto the private road leading to their summer home. Charlotte called out sharply to Bella and Kate. Both were trying to be the first to see the house by climbing onto the seat opposite.

"Sit properly," Charlotte said, "or you'll be like Humpty Dumpty!"

Bella and Kate reluctantly slumped down beside Min. "Humpty Dumpty fell off a wall," Bella pouted.

"You'll fall off the carriage," said Charlotte. "That's worse." She turned to her husband. "We must pay our respects to the Macdonalds. We should visit as soon as possible. Perhaps tomorrow?"

David nodded.

Donald Alexander Macdonald was a friend and associate of Charlotte's father, the Member for Glengarry in the House at Ottawa. His wife, Catherine, had died the previous year. Charlotte had sent a letter of condolence, but she and David had not been to Glengarry to express their sympathy in person.

"It must be especially difficult for Margaret Josephine," said Charlotte.

"How old is the girl?" David asked.

Charlotte thought a moment. "Sixteen? No, fifteen." She thought back to the death of her own mother when she was just half that age. "So very young to lose her mother."

Bella cried out and pointed. Standing out amongst the treetops, just beyond a far bend in the road, were the gingerbread peaks of the summer house.

Charlotte's father arrived from Ottawa the day after the House recessed until the fall. She and David were playing croquet with Bella and Kate on the broad lawn that lay between the house and the beach. Offshore, sailboats bobbed about, and a heavily laden trader rode low in the water where the river widened into Lake St. Francis.

When Bella and Kate saw their grandfather they dropped their mallets and ran to him. He bent to embrace them, but his eyes were fixed on his daughter. Charlotte thought she had never seen him look so forbidding. Bella tugged at her grandfather's hand.

"Come and play croquet with us!"

"Not just now," Joseph said. Then to Charlotte, "I would like to have a word with you."

"Yes, Father."

Charlotte and David exchanged a glance. They had agreed that when Joseph arrived, she should speak with him privately.

"Come along, children," said David. He put an arm around each of his daughters, firmly herding them towards the house.

"We'll see if Grandmother Whitehead can find us some raspberry cordial."

"Are you coming, Grandfather?" Bella called back over her shoulder.

"In a moment," said Joseph.

He waited until David and the children were out of earshot. Then he took Charlotte's letter from the inside pocket of his suitcoat and held it up to her.

"I have read this over several times," he said. "I would like an explanation."

O Lord, Charlotte thought in quick petition, help me make

him understand! Aloud she said, "I explained myself as well as I could." She hoped to make her point without seeming bold. "You must realize, Father, I did not decide this lightly. I have given it a great deal of thought."

"Rubbish!" Joseph stuffed the letter back in his pocket.

"I realize it is difficult for you," said Charlotte. "I can't help that, Father. My mind is made up."

Joseph studied his daughter. As much as her letter, and now this confrontation, distressed him, he admired her resolve. She reminded him of her mother, Isabella; a little of Margaret, too. Why in the world, he asked himself, do I always surround myself with strong-willed women?

"Does David know of this foolishness?" he finally asked. "Did you bully him as you are trying to bully me?"

Charlotte coloured. "I did not have to bully him, as you put it. He respects my right to do this."

"And your stepmother? Have you told her?"

"I have. She thinks as David does."

Charlotte's father fell silent.

"I did not give you every possible advantage," he said finally, "for you to work with sick and diseased people. For God's sake, Charlotte, have you any idea what you're getting into?"

"I have."

"It's morally wrong. God did not intend women to practise medicine."

"I don't believe that, Father. I don't believe you do, either."

From the back of the house they heard the housegirl call out to one of the children and the screen door slam shut.

"I might disown you," said Joseph. "Perhaps that would bring you to your senses."

Charlotte shook her head. "You would never do that, Father."

"Don't be too sure," said Joseph.

He turned his back on her. As he walked towards the house, Charlotte wanted to run after him. Instead she watched him reach the screened veranda, slowly mount the steps and disappear inside. She wondered why she felt such a sense of loss when she had plainly won.

Later that afternoon the family sat down to an early supper. Charlotte soon realized how wise she had been to make an ally of her stepmother. Whatever Margaret had said to Joseph, he gave no sign there had been words between father and daughter on the croquet pitch. He stood at the head of the refectory table by the window that looked out over Lake St. Francis and served cold cuts. While he layered slices on plates that the housegirl placed in front of him, he held forth on Manitoba's impending entry into Confederation.

"In less than a fortnight it's official," he said. "All that stands in the way is the half-breed Riel and his rebels."

"Does the prime minister think there will be bloodshed?" asked David.

Joseph shrugged. "Colonel Wolseley and sixteen hundred militiamen are on the march now to Fort Garry. I doubt Riel will stand and fight."

"Thank heavens!" said his wife. "Then that might be the end of it!"

It was while they were putting the children to bed that Charlotte got her first chance to ask Margaret what she had said to mollify Joseph.

"I explained your point of view as well as I could," she said. "I'm afraid your father still finds it unacceptable."

Charlotte frowned. "He seemed all right at supper."

Margaret brushed this aside. "Let me finish. I also told him that knowing you both as I do, I didn't expect either to give ground. You're very much alike, you know. After we talked for a while, your father came to terms with the situation. He does not want bad blood between himself and his only daughter."

"Then he's accepted my decision?"

Margaret shook her head. "Not exactly. He prefers to ignore it. If I were you, I would not discuss it with him further. I would simply go to Philadelphia."

This was less than Charlotte had hoped for, but she realized it was also more than it might have been. She thanked her stepmother for her support. She consoled herself with the thought that if she did not have her father's blessing, at least she had his forbearance.

Neither Charlotte nor her father discussed the matter again.

The day after their arrival, Charlotte and David had gone by carriage to Alexandria and paid their respects to Donald Macdonald and Margaret Josephine. On their return through Lancaster they had dropped in on David's cousin. Donald Ross

Dingwall had come to Canada from Hallkirk, Scotland, the previous fall. Before going on to Glengarry he had stayed a while with the Rosses in Côte des Neiges. His family had arranged for him to apprentice with an uncle, Peter McLeod, who was a successful jeweller in Lancaster.

Charlotte sympathized with the young Scot who was living so far from home and the Macdonald girl, who had lost her mother. On weekends when David came down from Montreal, she entertained for them. Sometimes Margaret Josephine arrived with Dr. Hingston, who was a frequent house guest of her father. They all passed the summer pleasantly, boating on Lake St. Francis, playing croquet or battledore and shuttlecock, and picnicking with the children by the riverbank. Charlotte spent much of her time with Bella, Kate and Min. Each passing day made her more conscious of how soon she would have to leave them. Sitting on the veranda one evening just before the children's bedtime, with Joseph and Margaret nearby, Charlotte carefully tried to explain to the children why she had to go to Philadelphia. Joseph got up and went inside.

Just before noon on the day before the House ended its summer recess, the carriage was brought around. It was already loaded with Joseph's luggage, ready to take him to the railway station in Lancaster. His family gathered at the front of the house to see him off. Joseph embraced his wife and his three grandchildren. He glanced at his daughter and looked away. Then he got into the carriage. Charlotte did not hold back. She felt that however valid she thought her point of view was, and her father his, they could not part like this. Out of the corner of his eye, as he pulled the carriage door shut, Joseph caught her movement forward. In the few quick steps it took her to reach the carriage he leaned over its side, awkwardly returning her embrace.

"I won't be seeing you at Christmas?" Joseph said.

"No. Not until some time after March."

Joseph nodded. "You take good care of yourself." His voice was gruffly demanding. "Don't forget to write."

"I won't, Father."

Joseph nodded again. He told the houseman to drive on, and the carriage clattered up the road. His answering wave to the children's shouted goodbyes was lost behind a tall stand of birch.

The weeks following the family's return to Montreal were busy ones for Charlotte. She had much to do for David and the children and to prepare herself to spend almost six months in Philadelphia. While her classes did not begin until early October, she wanted a week or so to get acquainted with her new surroundings. David offered to escort her, but since this would keep him from the children and from his work she convinced him it was better that she go alone. As much as she would miss her husband, Charlotte knew that it would be most difficult to part with the children. Bella had turned eight in June. She would have her schoolwork and friends to take her mind off her mother's absence. Kate, who would be five on the last day of September, and Min, just three in mid-October, would be home all day. When she let herself think about it, Charlotte was disturbed that she would miss both her younger daughters' birthdays. It would be the first time.

On the eve of her departure, Charlotte and David retired early. Charlotte's feelings were mixed. She had misgivings over leaving David and the children. At the same time, she was excited at the prospect of a new and compelling adventure. Sometimes she felt as much an enigma to herself as she knew she was to her father. She watched from beneath the bedclothes as David got into his nightshirt and blew out the lamp. They lay in the darkness for a while, neither of them speaking. Charlotte thought again how remarkably understanding her husband was.

"I'll miss you," she said.

"And I you."

"It will seem longer than it really is."

"Yes."

"But not too long."

David remained silent. Charlotte felt his hand seeking hers. She reached out and touched him.

Immediately after luncheon the next day, Charlotte prepared to leave for the railway station. She fussed over the children, telling them things they had heard repeatedly over the previous few days as though they had just occurred to her. They were to listen to their grandfather and grandmother Ross and do what they were told. . . . They were to eat everything that was put in front of them. . . . They were to go to bed without having to be told more than once. Finally the list became so long, and David knew they had heard it so often anyway, that he hustled his wife out the door and into the waiting carriage. Even then, with her three daughters standing by their grandparents, Charlotte called out instructions to them: Bella was to study hard in school; . . . she and Kate were to help care for their younger sister. . . . David lurched the carriage forward.

Charlotte was silent while her husband drove along the Tollgate Road to Montreal, mentally going over the preparations she had made for her departure. By the time they passed the toll booth, she had satisfied herself that she had done all she could to leave her family well-organized. It had not been easy for her. She had gone over all the clothing her husband and children would wear from fall through to spring, making sure everything was in good repair. She had replaced articles David had outworn or she thought soon would, and the children had outgrown. It had taken several weeks of mending and shopping. As usual, Charlotte had been able to rely on Bella to look after herself and her two sisters.

"Bless Bella," she said to David. "She's such a help."

David nodded. He gave the horse loose rein, knowing it knew the way from the house in Côte des Neiges to downtown Montreal as well as he did.

"She's going to miss you," said David. "I remember the morning we saw you off at the station and she cried out to go."

"I'd forgotten."

"She looked the same when you left the house."

"She'll get over it," Charlotte said. "She has you and her

sisters, as well as her school friends. Bella's well able to look after herself, as young as she is."

Shortly before half past three, David put Charlotte aboard one of the luxurious sleeping and dining carriages that were called Pullman palace cars. He had delivered her trunk to the baggage master earlier that week. He escorted her to her seat and placed her hand luggage in the overhead rack. Then he leaned over and gave her a quick embrace.

"You'll be sure and write as soon as you're settled?"

Charlotte smiled up at him. "The first moment I have to myself."

"If you need anything you'll let me know?"

"I will. Don't worry, I'll be just fine."

He straightened up in the aisle. "Well, goodbye then."

"Goodbye. Look after yourself and the children."

"I will."

"Be sure and give them my love."

David nodded. He left the car, stopping on the station platform by her window to exchange a wave and a smile. When he was gone, Charlotte took her railway ticket from her handbag. She examined it curiously. It would take seven different railways, a ferryboat and almost twenty-five hours for her to reach her destination. She put her ticket back in her handbag and set about making herself comfortable.

CHAPTER ❦ SIX

Philadelphia, Fall, 1870

*T*HE TWO QUAKER WOMEN were waiting with a liveryman on the platform of the west Philadelphia terminal when Charlotte stepped down from the railway carriage. She recognized them immediately. Her stepmother had told her to look for two elderly ladies in the wide-brimmed hats with gathered crown and drab brown dresses worn by the Religious Society of Friends.

"Aunt Annie! Aunt Johan!" Charlotte called out. She waved to identify herself as well as to attract their attention.

The two women responded with an exchange of pleased smiles, and hurried up the station platform. Their liveryman followed, detouring to where the railway porter was unloading the passengers' hand luggage.

"Charlotte Ross!" Johan greeted her. She reached out and took one of Charlotte's hands in both of hers. "My sister and I welcome thee to Philadelphia!"

The sisters lived in the eighteen-hundred block on Ridge Avenue in a comfortable, two-storey house that was typical of upper-middle-class neighbourhoods in Philadelphia. Margaret had written to them on Charlotte's behalf asking if they would be agreeable to having her as a guest in their home. Their reply had been promptly affirmative. In the exchange of letters that followed, the sisters had refused at first to accept payment. Charlotte had insisted. They finally had settled on four dollars a week for room and board – two dollars less than the going rate for women students. Even at that, the sisters had felt compelled to assure her that no more comfortable room could be found at any price in all Philadelphia.

Charlotte was pleased to find this to be true. Equally important, the house was within easy walking distance of Woman's Medical College. Over tea and cakes in the parlour she satisfied their polite curiosity about herself and members of the McDonald family who had migrated north to Canada almost fifty years earlier.

The liveryman had delivered Charlotte's trunk and hand luggage to the upstairs room the sisters had prepared for her. As she unpacked, neatly folding and placing her things in bureau drawers, she reflected on Aunt Johan and Aunt Annie. They had agreed that while Charlotte was not actually a relative, this was as good a way as any for her to address them. She was also getting used to their use of *thee* and *thy* for *you* and *your*. She knew this to be the Quaker manner of speaking.

Something else had puzzled Charlotte from the outset. She said she thought the sisters would have been surprised by her reason for wishing to come to Philadelphia. They were amused.

"The Friends believe in equality," said Johan. "We were

active abolitionists before the Civil War ended slavery five years ago. Now we seek prison reform, like our English friend, Elizabeth Fry."

"And equal rights for women," said Annie. "It was the Friends who helped found the school thee will attend."

Believing that women were as entitled as men to advanced education and a profession, five of the six men on the first faculty had been Quakers.

There was still an hour or so before dinner. Charlotte was eager to see where she would study for the next three years. She set off to walk the four blocks from the sisters' house to North College Avenue.

What she found was a disappointment. Woman's Medical College of Pennsylvania was not a place, as she had expected, but only a name. Before her stood the Woman's Hospital of Philadelphia, a squat brick building of uncertain parentage; the sire was perhaps gingerbread Gothic and the dam early American armoury. Charlotte found nothing to please the eye about or around it. Other than a small protest of grass, there was not a green thing between the building and the black iron railing that fenced it from the hitching posts and gas lamp standards of the sidewalk.

Charlotte was thoughtful on the walk back to Ridge Avenue. The other institution of learning in her life had been the Convent of the Sacred Heart, with its shining cupolas and cross-topped spire rising above tall trees and landscaped grounds. As she turned onto the walk to the sisters' house, she decided in retrospect that her surroundings did not count. It was the dream and not the place that had brought her here to Philadelphia.

That evening Charlotte wrote these and other thoughts in a rambling letter to David. She added personal postscripts to each of her three children. She also intended to write to her father and Margaret, but she found the long trip and the excitement of her arrival more tiring than she had realized. She undressed slowly. She liked the sisters and her lodgings, which were just as comfortable as she was accustomed to at home. When she had put on her nightdress, she turned down the gas lamp and got into bed. She was already asleep when one of the sisters looked in on her a few minutes later. Johan's sympathetic smile for the tired traveller was lost in the darkness. She closed the door again as gently as Charlotte would have shut it on one of her own sleeping daughters.

"Welcome to the twenty-first session of the Woman's Medical College of Pennsylvania, the oldest woman's medical school in the world!"

The speaker was Dr. Ann Preston, one of its early graduates. As well as being dean of studies, she was professor of physiology and hygiene. Dean Preston was delivering the welcoming address to students in the lecture room of Woman's Hospital.

Charlotte looked around her at the other students. All wore the starched white shirtwaists, full black skirts and high-button shoes that would be their uniform for the next three years. Each had her hair tied back in a severe bun. Charlotte exchanged a tentative smile with a woman who would be one of her classmates.

"This college was founded twenty years ago," Dean Preston was saying. "From its humble beginnings and small enrolment I now see before me fifty-seven young ladies. I am proud to announce that this represents the largest number of students in our history!"

When the applause had ended, she described how the school had been begun in a house in a residential neighbourhood. Its short but continuous history since then had been broken by only one year, during the Civil War. She spoke about the difficulties it had overcome, first just to survive, then to grow to its present record enrolment as part of Woman's Hospital. Over the years, early graduates like herself and women doctors from elsewhere had gradually made it possible for the faculty of eight to be made up equally of men and women.

"Women still face formidable obstacles to higher education," said Dean Preston. "This is particularly true of you who have chosen to study towards a doctorate in medicine. You will find that you not only have to work as hard as your male counterparts," she warned, "but harder. You will not only have to be as good, but better."

She waited for the low murmur from among the students to subside.

"There are three ladies among you from countries other than the United States. I would ask you to please stand as you are introduced."

Dean Preston glanced down at a page on the lectern. "Caroline Hamlin, from Constantinople, Turkey. Charlotte Yhlen, Helsingborg, Sweden. Charlotte Ross, from Montreal, Canada."

Charlotte stood up, feeling as awkward as the other two at being singled out, but managing a smile at the applause that followed the introductions.

The dean waited until they were seated again and the room was silent. "To all of you ladies," she said brusquely, "welcome to the study of medicine!"

Charlotte and her classmates met in the secretary of the faculty's office after the opening ceremony with Dr. Cleveland, who was also professor of obstetrics and diseases of women. She went over lists of required textbooks with them and worked out timetables. Some of the first-year students had questions to ask. One of them was having difficulty finding lodgings. Dr. Cleveland produced a listing of suitable ones at different prices. Then she gave them the rest of the day to shop for textbooks, notepads, pens, pencils and whatever else they needed. As Charlotte left the office, she was approached by a classmate she recognized as another foreign student.

"Apparently we are namesakes," the woman said, her English accented. "I am Charlotte Yhlen, from Helsingborg."

Charlotte returned her smile. "Charlotte Ross."

"You are from Canada?"

"Yes. Montreal."

"We have some things in common besides our first name," said the Swedish girl. She grinned. "Cold winters, for one. And another, our wish to become doctors."

Both Charlottes, like the rest of their classmates, found they had time for little more than hallway friendships in the weeks that followed. Classes were from ten o'clock in the morning to six o'clock in the afternoon, with a short break for luncheon. On Saturdays they ended four hours earlier, but without a noon break. There were no classes on the Sabbath. Every night reminded Charlotte of those she had spent in her father's home in Clinton, studying medical books by lamplight while she looked after Mary Anne. Sometimes she did not get to bed until it seemed almost pointless, when the pale rose of the Philadelphia dawn was already beginning to unfold outside her bedroom window.

The strain of such long hours of lectures and home study on Charlotte and her classmates was not lost on the members of the faculty. Dr. Cleveland in particular was concerned. A month after the start of the winter exercises, she mentioned it in a Monday morning assembly in the lecture room.

"I'm sure many of you are having difficulty in keeping up with your studies," she said. "We on the faculty appreciate this. Beginning next fall the session will be extended two full weeks, from the present twenty to twenty-two." She paused. "Dean Preston and I are worried that some of you may suffer ill effects from putting in so much work over such a short period."

There was a murmur of approval. Some of the students exchanged an exaggerated look of relief, which Dr. Cleveland acknowledged with a smile.

"It's a little soon for that," she said. "The extension will not take effect until next fall. Until then, your schedules will remain the same. As you leave, I will provide timetables for the clinics we have arranged for you at three other hospitals."

Charlotte and her classmates were looking forward to these twice-weekly clinics. They were to be held at Pennsylvania Hospital, which was famous for advances in the treatment of industrial accidents; Wills' Ophthalmic, specializing in eye care and surgery; and Philadelphia Hospital, one of the country's largest general hospitals.

As the students left the lecture room, Dr. Cleveland handed out the timetables. When it came Charlotte's turn, the dean asked her to remain after the others. Early in the session, Dr. Cleveland had seen in Charlotte the same qualities that had impressed her teachers at the Convent of the Sacred Heart. When everyone else had gone, Dr. Cleveland gathered up her papers and walked with Charlotte to the door.

"I've been reviewing your work, Mrs. Ross," she said. "You're doing quite well."

"Thank you, Dr. Cleveland."

"Do you find it difficult to keep up with your classes and the study time involved?"

"Like my classmates," Charlotte admitted, "I am kept busy."

"Well, take care you don't overdo it."

84

Although she recognized this as just a reference to her hours of home study, Dr. Cleveland's remark startled Charlotte. More than two months had passed since David had made love to her on the night before she left for Philadelphia. She had little doubt now that she was with child.

On the following Wednesday, Charlotte and her classmates attended the first of the clinics at Philadelphia Hospital. An earlier clinic was still in progress when they arrived. They waited outside in the corridor. As women students, they took their clinics separately from the men. The arrangement was intended both to save any embarrassment that might arise from a mixed class and to avoid possible harassment. In its first twenty years, Woman's Medical College had succeeded in overcoming much of the prejudice shown by many members of the medical profession and the Philadelphia community. Despite this, it was still common for some of the men students to jeer at the women as they left the clinics, sometimes bombarding them with spitballs. Everyone knew of at least one classmate who had been spat on – staining both her pride and her crisp white shirtwaist with tobacco juice.

When the door to the clinic opened, a class of young men spilled out. They were laughing and talking until they saw the women students. Charlotte felt that she and her classmates were as conspicuous as penguins in their black skirts and white shirtwaists. The first few young men fell silent, then those behind them. As they walked past, some nodded uncertainly. Others stared with frank curiosity, looking back over their shoulders. One whispered something to another and they broke into muffled laughter. Charlotte felt someone brush by and breathe into her ear.

"Slut."

She glanced back at him, startled. He was a pleasant-looking young man, not much older than her brother William. He walked on as though nothing had been said. Charlotte felt a hot flush in her cheeks. No one had ever spoken to her like that before. Her embarrassment gave way to anger.

"Charlotte?"

She turned at the sound of Charlotte Yhlen's voice.

"Is anything wrong?"

She caught hold of herself and shook her head. "No. No, nothing's wrong."

"Come on, then. They'll close the door on us."

Charlotte looked once more up the corridor. It was empty now and silent. She went with her friend into the clinic.

On their first day, Dean Preston had warned the assembled students that they would have to work harder and be better because they were women challenging in a profession dominated by men. As the weeks wore on, Charlotte and her classmates learned to appreciate what she had meant. Their lives seemed to be one continuous round of lectures and study, with precious little time left over for eating and sleeping.

Three days before the Christmas break, Charlotte lost her baby.

She had been overworking herself, she knew. She had ignored Dr. Cleveland's advice, who was not even aware that she was pregnant, as well as her own experience that she did not carry babies easily. She was in her room, studying late into the night by the light of the gas lamp. She felt it first as a sharp stitch in her side, which went away as quickly as it had come. She was again bent over her books when a spasm made her cry out and clutch at herself with both hands. She got up and stumbled to the door, feeling a warm wetness in her nightdress. She managed to get the door open and call out before she began falling. She heard her own voice and Johan's from down the hallway. Then she felt herself falling faster and farther. As much as she tried to reach out and grasp Dr. Cleveland's hand, she could not keep herself from going away.

CHAPTER SEVEN

Philadelphia, Fall, 1871

*C*HARLOTTE RETURNED to Philadelphia two days before the start of the twenty-second session. She now realized that, in the three months before she was forced to leave the previous year, she had been much lonelier than she had let on, even to herself. She particularly had missed the children. When she applied in mid-summer to be re-admitted to first year, she already had decided to bring Kate and Min with her to Philadelphia.

Most of Charlotte's family opposed her return to her studies. Her father in particular read into his daughter's collapse what he had known all along – that as a woman she was emotionally and physically incapable of coping with the stress involved in the study and practice of medicine. David disagreed with Joseph. Concerned as he was with Charlotte's well-being, he considered her father's assessment unfair.

"Joseph's only half right," he said. "If Philadelphia's to blame it's only because the baby and your studies together proved too much for you. It's not the first time you've had difficulty getting through the early months," he reminded her. "If you're as determined as ever to study to be a doctor, you'll get no opposition from me."

This had proved to be David's last word on the matter. Only Charlotte knew how deeply disappointed he was at the loss of what might have been a son.

It was agreed that Bella would remain in Montreal with her father and grandparents. The two younger children would accompany their mother to Philadelphia. David's brother had a daughter, Edith, who had finished school in June. She was eager to go along as a companion to her aunt Charlotte and her two cousins. Accommodations were no problem. Johan and Annie had written Charlotte saying that her niece and the two children were as welcome at the Ridge Avenue house as she was herself.

"God bless you both," Charlotte had thought aloud on reading their letter. It had removed the last obstacle to resuming her studies.

The return to Philadelphia was like a homecoming. Johan and Annie outdid the welcome promised in their letter, fussing like grandmothers over Charlotte, her niece and her two daughters. Edith unpacked their hand luggage and trunks, getting well-meant, if questionable, help from Kate and Min. Charlotte and the sisters talked about the night the previous winter when Johan had heard Charlotte's cries and found her collapsed in the hallway.

"And thee are feeling none the worse now?" Johan asked, while Annie refilled their tea cups.

"Just as though it never happened," Charlotte reassured her.

"Good. Thee are a healthy young woman, Charlotte. Thee have time enough to give thy husband a son."

Charlotte hid her amusement behind a sip of tea. She had learned from living with David that Scottish people are outspoken about their priorities. It was obvious that the sisters had made hers the continued pursuit of her medical studies. When they had finished tea, Charlotte helped her niece install the four of them in two upstairs bedrooms. Edith shared the larger one with Kate and Min. Then she took the children out to play. Charlotte set off to walk the six blocks to Woman's Hospital.

When she entered the office of the secretary of the faculty, Charlotte again experienced a sense of homecoming. Dr. Cleveland was seated at her desk. She was going over the second-year students' timetable with Charlotte Yhlen. Charlotte and the young Swedish woman exclaimed their pleasure at meeting again, both trying to get in the first word until they broke off, laughing.

"Welcome back," Dr. Cleveland said, rising.

"I'm glad to be back," Charlotte assured her.

Dr. Cleveland had written Charlotte soon after she had been forced to give up her studies and return to Montreal. She had written again when Charlotte was summering at Glengarry.

"I want to thank you for your encouraging letters," said Charlotte. "They meant much to me."

"I knew you were terribly disappointed," Dr. Cleveland replied. "I thought my writing might help."

"Your letters did." She turned to her Swedish friend. "Yours did, too. It was very thoughtful of both of you."

"We were concerned," said Charlotte Yhlen.

"As I mentioned in my replies, there were complications. I had plenty of time convalescing to get used to the idea of starting all over again. That vexed me, of course. I hated the thought of being set back a whole year." She made a face at Charlotte Yhlen. "I still envy you your whole year ahead of me!"

"Put your setbacks to work for you," said Dr. Cleveland. "Think of yourself as having a head start on the rest of the first-year class."

"I'll try to remember that," Charlotte said.

They talked for a while about the previous year's enrolment and how many were returning. Seventeen third-year students, all of them Americans, had graduated the previous March. A few others, either from the pressures of study or for some other reason, would not be back. Among these was Caroline Hamlin, the Turkish woman from Constantinople. Even so, Dr. Cleveland was quick to point out, there were fifty-eight registrations for the twenty-second session, one more than in the preceding year. Charlotte and her Swedish friend were two of only three students from outside the United States. The third, Dr. Cleveland advised them with a glance at the registry, was Emma Palmer, from London, England.

One of the requirements for graduation was the writing of a thesis in the final year. The subject was up to the student. Thinking back to what Dr. Cleveland had said about putting your setbacks to work for you, Charlotte had already decided on the subject of hers.

The addition of two weeks to the length of the session, without any increase in lectures and clinics, gave the students some time to themselves. Before this extension they had found they quite literally had none. Now they still studied late nights and Saturdays, but if their work was caught up they could afford the luxury of a leisurely Sunday.

After church services on what looked to be the last warm afternoon in late fall, Charlotte went on a picnic with Edith and the two children. Fairmount Park was a popular site for strollers and picnickers on the banks of the Schuylkill River. It was easy to reach by horse car, and pretty enough with its grassy slopes and meadows, though so logged out in previous years that it was sparsely treed. Charlotte wrote David about the picnic and the park in her next letter home. She wrote every week, always adding a brief personal note to Bella. Sometimes when she was so tired from study that she had difficulty sleeping, Charlotte questioned herself for not being with her eldest daughter. Even though she knew Bella was self-reliant beyond her nine years, their separation troubled her. It made Charlotte uncomfortably mindful of how she had suffered through the loss of her own mother when she was not much younger. But, invariably in the mornings, her feeling of guilt was lost in her concentration on another day's studies and the challenge of succeeding.

Charlotte also wrote regularly to her father and stepmother. Joseph's replies both saddened and amused her. He ignored her circumstances and whereabouts, his only concession being to the envelope, which required her address in Philadelphia. In a letter he wrote not long after she resumed her studies, he announced an end to his career in federal politics.

> As a condition to British Columbia becoming our sixth province, the Prime Minister is politically committed to building a national railroad.
>
> I will not be among those seeking re-election next year. I can't imagine myself sitting through five more years of watching the Prime Minister run this country as conductor, stoker and engineman, all in one. When my term is up, I intend to go back to doing what I do best, which is building railroads.

In mid-November, Sarah Hale invited Charlotte to Thanksgiving dinner. After taking the Ridge Avenue horse car into the business and shopping district of old Philadelphia, Charlotte had dropped by the Chestnut Street offices of *Godey's Lady's Book*. Now eighty-three, Sarah Hale was still editor of the most successful fashion and family magazine in America. She had been pleased to extend her invitation to Charlotte Yhlen and Emma Palmer.

Sarah Hale lived with her daughter Frances and son-in-law, Dr. Louis Boudinot Hunter, a retired naval surgeon who now had a flourishing practice in Philadelphia. A hackney carriage had been sent for their three dinner guests. On the ride to the house, the carriage and pair clip-clopping along pavingstone streets, Charlotte talked with her two friends about Sarah Hale. They already knew, from her editorials, of her outspoken views on women's rights and responsibilities. They were looking forward to meeting her.

"You will find her a fascinating person," said Charlotte. "It was she who convinced President Lincoln to declare this day a national holiday."

"You're not serious!" said Emma Palmer.

Charlotte was amused by her English friend's scepticism. "Ask her yourself," she said with a laugh.

Emma thought that if the occasion arose she would. As the hackney turned onto Locust Street, she tried to imagine a magazine editor exercising the same influence on Queen Victoria. She could not.

The Hunter house was on one of the straight and narrow streets that had been laid out like a checkerboard by founder William Penn. When the hackney stopped, the front door opened and Dr. Hunter emerged. He greeted Charlotte and her two friends warmly, giving each his arm in turn as they stepped down from the carriage. His wife, Frances, received their guests in the front hall. When the introductions had been made, Dr. Hunter assisted them with their coats. Then he ushered them into the sitting room. His wife went to see what was keeping her mother.

As Charlotte had promised, Sarah Hale was not a disappointment to Charlotte Yhlen and Emma Palmer. She made a dramatic entrance, her head in a coiffed silver cloud over her customary costume of mourning black. Her daughter introduced

Charlotte's two friends. Sarah Hale took each by the hand. Then she walked to a wing chair by the fireplace and sat down.

"I understand you are classmates of Charlotte's," she said.

Charlotte Yhlen let Emma Palmer reply. "Yes, ma'am."

"Are you finding your studies difficult?"

"Very!"

Vigorous nods from other two guests served to make this unanimous.

"Nothing worth doing is easily done," said Sarah Hale. "I admire you three helping show the way to others. God bless you for it."

Sarah Hale glanced at her son-in-law. He was standing over an iron poker he had placed in the glowing coals of the fireplace.

"Would you agree, Louis?" She looked back to their guests. "My daughter's husband is not one of those who hold that women have no place in medicine."

"Quite so," said Dr. Hunter. "While the notion is not popular among most of my colleagues, some of us do see the need for women doctors."

Sarah Hale winked at their guests. "Surgeons, too?"

Dr. Hunter knew when his leg was being pulled. "I frankly should hate the competition," he said, keeping a straight face. "Especially from such a comely quarter."

Sarah Hale clapped her hands. She was as delighted with their guests' failure to look properly demure at this as she was with her son-in-law's reply. Although Dr. Hunter had made light of it, they all knew that while some of the resistance to women doctors was based on moral grounds, or questions of emotional and physical makeup, most came from those who saw medicine as an exclusive and profitable men's club and wished to keep it that way.

Sarah Hale was still chuckling when her daughter brought her husband a filled pewter jug from the kitchen. Dr. Hunter took the poker cherry red from the fire. He thrust it into the pitcher, mulling the wine punch with a guttural hiss that translated instantly into a pungent cloud of steam. He poured the hot punch into miniatures of the pot-bellied pitcher. While his wife served them from a pewter tray, Emma Palmer seized on the opportunity to ask about the Thanksgiving holiday.

Sarah Hale glanced at Charlotte. "You told her about that, did you?" She smiled in reminiscence. "Thanksgiving was always our most important feast in New England. This was because it began there, in Massachusetts, with the landing of the Pilgrims at Plymouth Rock." She sipped her punch. "I'd been trying for years to get that blessed event the recognition it deserved. Talking about it. Writing editorials. Finally, I went to see Mr. Lincoln."

"When was that?" asked Emma.

"Seven years ago. The year before he was assassinated. We talked a long while and in the end he agreed with me. Soon after, he declared Thanksgiving a national holiday, the fourth Thursday in November."

Dr. Hunter raised his mug. "A toast," he said. "To Mister Lincoln, Mother Hale and the good Pilgrims of Plymouth Rock!"

Christmas came and went. Winter succumbed to the insistence of spring. Charlotte and her two friends were among those granted their year at commencement exercises held in mid-March at Philadelphia's Musical Fund Hall. A month later, Charlotte and her husband were luncheon guests of her younger brother at Montreal's most fashionable hotel. William had invited them to dine with him to meet a friend. At the time, David had mentioned to Charlotte that her brother had met a girl in Montreal while she had been in Philadelphia.

"Do I know her?" Charlotte had asked.

"I don't think so. Her name is Caroline. Caroline Nicholson."

William would be twenty-three in August. He had completed his apprenticeship with Watts and Co. and now was a practising pharmacist in Toronto. Charlotte realized that despite this she still thought of him as the little brother she had left behind in Clinton six years earlier, when she and David had moved to Montreal.

On the ride in from Côte des Neiges, she wondered aloud about William's intentions. "Do you think he's serious about this girl?"

David shrugged. "Who's to say? He's still a young man, but he's been to Montreal more often in three months than over the past three years."

He reined up at the tollgate. "He said he might move here." David grinned. "I told him if he intended to keep seeing the Nicholson girl he'd save a pretty penny in train fares."

He started up the horse again with a light flick of the reins.

"How old is she?" asked Charlotte.

"I'd say about nineteen. No more."

"Is she pretty?"

David looked mildly amused. "You know your brother William."

St. Lawrence Hall was on St. James Street, convenient both to shopping and to Montreal's financial district. As the *maître d'* seated them at their table, Charlotte realized that this was something more than just a casual foursome. William clearly had planned the luncheon to introduce his sister and her husband to someone he looked upon as very special. Charlotte took an immediate liking to the young woman seated opposite her. Conversation between them came easily.

"It has been eleven years since I was last here," said Charlotte. "My father came for me at the Convent of the Sacred Heart. We stayed at this hotel overnight. We caught the train for home the next morning."

The waiter took their order and the menus.

"The Prince of Wales was here to open Victoria Bridge," Charlotte continued. "He and his entourage stayed at this hotel."

The bridge had established a vital link with the United States, connecting Montreal by rail with the Eastern Seaboard.

Peter Nicholson, Caroline's father, was the contractor who had built it.

"Did you like the convent?" asked Caroline.

"As a student, very much," said Charlotte. "The nuns and the lay teachers were all excellent. The father of the young girl who sang for the Prince of Wales at the bridge opening taught voice. Her name was Marie Louise Lajeunesse. Today she's a world-famous concert soprano. Madame Albani?"

"Of course!" exclaimed Caroline. "Were you classmates?"

Charlotte shook her head. "I was sixteen. She was much younger. I think perhaps eight or nine. Even at that age, she was always on stage. She got so wrought up playing the part of the devil at our graduation-day tableau that she became hysterical. She had to be put to bed."

Caroline looked sympathetic. "Poor child!" she said. "What part did you play?"

Charlotte sighed. "Because I was not a Catholic, some of the nuns insisted I could not be a saint. Marie Louise had already been given the part of the devil. I was heartbroken."

"What a shame!"

"Sister Trincano, the mother superior, found a solution. She said that since there were no religious differences in heaven, I could be an angel."

"How very wise of her!"

"Yes, said Charlotte. I've always thought, as well, how very Christian."

By the time the waiter returned, the two women had set a day the following week to meet at Victoria Square, outside Henry Morgan and Co., to do the shops together. When Charlotte got home later that day there was a letter waiting for her from Philadelphia. Dr. Cleveland had become as much her friend as her professor over the previous two years. They corresponded regularly. David saw his wife frown as she read the letter.

"Dean Preston is dead," she said finally. "She passed away on the eighteenth."

Charlotte handed him the first of the neatly scripted note pages. "You've heard me speak of her. She was one of the early graduates."

David read the page and handed it back to her. "Did you know Dr. Preston well?" he asked gently.

"All of the students did," said Charlotte. "She was one of us. She never stopped facing up to those who opposed women doctors."

On a morning early in September, Charlotte sat down at the writing desk in her bedroom. David had left for work. Bella and Kate were at school. Min was being of dubious help to the housegirl, who was putting up preserves in the summer kitchen. Charlotte thoughtfully touched the tip of the penholder to her teeth, her elbow resting on the desk by a sheet of letter paper. Outside her bedroom window, an anxious robin tweaked the branch of an early turning maple. She watched for a moment and then it was gone. Charlotte reluctantly returned to the blank page. She dipped the nib of her pen in ink and began her letter.

Montreal, Canada
September 10, 1872

Dear Dr. Cleveland:

It is with deep regret that I must advise you that I will not be returning for the twenty-third session this fall. I am again with child and do not feel in good conscience that I can risk yet another miscarriage, to which, as you know, I am all too readily susceptible.

Please give my best wishes to Charlotte Yhlen and Anne Palmer when you see them, and to the rest of my classmates.

I look forward to resuming my studies at the start of the twenty-fourth session.

I will write at some length later. For now I must close, with the hope that this note finds you and those you hold dear in good health.

Charlotte

Charlotte's fourth daughter was born on Monday, March 10. Charlotte named her Edith Caroline Cleveland. She was to be called Carrie, after William's fiancée. The two women had become fast friends since the luncheon the previous spring at St. Lawrence Hall. The name Edith was for the niece who accompanied Charlotte and the children to Philadelphia; Cleveland was for the woman who had been named dean of the Woman's Medical College of Pennsylvania after the death of Dr. Preston.

Charlotte and her niece arrived in Philadelphia on the last day of September, two days before the start of the twenty-fourth session. They brought with them Min, who would be six in mid-October, and Carrie, going on seven months. Bella and Kate remained behind in Montreal with their father.

After everyone had settled in and she had traded news over tea with Johan and Annie, Charlotte wheeled the baby the short piece to Woman's Hospital. She was welcomed by Dr. Cleveland, who fussed over her namesake before bringing Charlotte up to date on her classmates. Her old friend Charlotte Yhlen had graduated the previous March and returned to Sweden.

"We had four ladies from Canada last session," said the new dean. "Only one, Jennifer Trout from Toronto, has returned. Perhaps you know her?"

Charlotte shook her head.

"Mrs. Trout came to us after spending a year at the Toronto School of Medicine. She told me that she and her classmate were the first two ladies to be admitted to a medical school in your country."

Charlotte was surprised. She had not been aware that any school had finally opened its doors to women. Why, then, had she come to Philadelphia?

"Did she say why she left?"

"She did," said Dr. Cleveland. "She said that she and her classmate could not put up with any more humiliation."

In the hallway after the opening ceremony, Charlotte met again with Emma Palmer. Her English friend was in her final year. They introduced themselves to Jennie Trout, who was standing speaking with another student, Emily Tefft, from upstate New York.

"Dr. Cleveland mentioned that you studied in Toronto," Charlotte said to Jennie.

"My friend Emily Stowe and I both did," she replied. "Emily graduated six years ago from the New York Medical College for Women. When she returned to Toronto, there was nowhere she could take the one session she needed at a Canadian school to be licensed."

"That's unfair!" exclaimed Emma.

"Worse than that," said Jennie. "Because she couldn't be licensed, she practised illegally. She was arrested and fined. Finally, last year, we were admitted to Toronto School."

"I'd say about time!" said Emma.

"It didn't end there. Being the first two women students, we were told that whatever happened we weren't to complain. We soon found out why. Our classmates, even some of the professors, made it clear we weren't welcome."

"How?" asked Charlotte.

"We were so badgered that we waited until class started to run in and take our seats. Then one day we found ourselves sitting on broken eggs. So many obscene pictures were drawn on the classroom walls that they had to be repainted. One professor amused himself and the class by telling lewd stories. Emily finally put an end to that by threatening to tell his wife."

"I'm surprised you put up with it as long as you did," said Charlotte.

"Well, we finally decided that we'd had enough. I applied here. Emily never did take the exam for her Ontario licence. She said they likely would have failed her anyway."

"What did she do?" asked Emma.

"She's gone back to practising without one."

No one spoke for a few moments. All four were thinking of the difficulties they and their classmates already had overcome and those they would surely have to face in the future. Charlotte thought back to the young man who had confronted her as she was entering the clinic on accidents at Pennsylvania Hospital.

"I can imagine how hard it must have been for you and your friend," she said to Jennie. "I was insulted at one of our clinics. I'd only been here a few weeks. As much as we were told to expect it, it still came as a shock."

Emma looked at her in surprise. "You never told me."

Charlotte shrugged. "I didn't think it was worth mentioning."

On the following Friday, Charlotte and her classmates were given their first lecture on physiology and hygiene by Dr. Henry Hartshorne. This had been Dr. Preston's subject when she was dean. After her death it was assigned to Dr. Hartshorne, who also taught hygiene and diseases of children.

Charlotte heard a low hiss behind her and looked over her shoulder at Emma. Her friend made a puzzled frown and nodded towards the entrance to the classroom. Dr. Hartshorne was pacing back and forth in the hallway, pausing at the doorway to look in, then abruptly disappearing again. Finally he entered, scowling, carrying a sheaf of papers at his side. He swung the door shut behind him and marched to the lectern. The class quieted. For a few moments he shuffled the papers, not looking up nor losing the scowl on his face.

"In this series of lectures," he said, "we will concern ourselves with the sciences of physiology and hygiene."

For what seemed to Charlotte a very long time he looked at the class and they at him. Then his whole manner became confused. He scooped up the papers from the lectern, wheeled, and stood with his back to them. "We will examine normal human functions and health through personal cleanliness."

Dr. Hartshorne said this so awkwardly that someone at the rear of the room giggled. If Dr. Hartshorne heard, he did not let on. He took a deep breath and launched into his lecture. He spoke so quickly that no one could take notes. A few tried, jotting down a word here and a phrase there, scribbling furiously. Finally they, too, gave up and just sat back and listened with the rest of the class.

The lecture was over. Dr. Hartshorne did an about turn, strode from the lectern and disappeared into the corridor.

There was a brief silence.

Then everyone began laughing and talking at once until someone finally called out that this was serious. The room silenced. Dr. Hartshorne's course was an important part of the curriculum. There was no telling when and if the bashful professor might face the class, and, more important still, speak slowly enough so that they could make notes.

"I have every word he said." The voice belonged to a young New England woman who was in her second year. "I know Mr. Pitman's shorthand."

Charlotte and the others spent their lunch break taking

notes. Dr. Hartshorne's lecture was read out to them by their classmate. She had learned stenography working in the Boston home office of her missionary father.

Charlotte and Jennie Trout were not close. Jennie spent most of her time with Emily Tefft, the student from New York. Charlotte did not feel as easy with either of them as she had from the beginning with Charlotte Yhlen and Emma Palmer. For one thing, they had quite different attitudes towards how to go about practising their profession after graduation.

Because Jennie had put in a session at Toronto School before coming to Philadelphia, she had already met one of the two requirements to being accepted by the Ontario College of Physicians and Surgeons. The other was to appear before the admissions board. Unlike Emily Stowe, who had disdained to take the all-male board's oral and written examinations, Jennie was prepared to do whatever was necessary to be licensed.

Charlotte was not. She felt that on graduation day she would have won her doctorate in medicine fairly and with it the right to practise. She did not feel obligated to put in another year's study under the demeaning conditions that Jennie and Emily had experienced at Toronto School. Besides, she wished to practise in Montreal, not Toronto. She had discussed this with Dr. Hingston, who was an influential member of the Quebec College. He had advised Charlotte, regretfully, that its members were not prepared to admit her, nor any woman, whatever special qualifications were met or examinations passed. Charlotte did not care. She had come to Philadelphia to learn medicine. She would return to Montreal to practise it.

The Twenty-First Annual Commencement was held in mid-March at Philadelphia's Horticultural Hall. For Charlotte it was a day of mixed emotions. For the second time she remained an undergraduate while a friend and former classmate mounted the podium to be awarded her doctorate. The previous year it had been Charlotte Yhlen. Now it was Emma Palmer. As happy as she was for both her old friends, Charlotte was dejected all over again that she had had to withdraw from her first year and absent herself from her third. She was also more than a little depressed at having to spend an additional ten weeks in Philadelphia working on her preceptorship. This was the part of their training that was actual practice, under an approved doctor or at a hospital. It meant that she would not be rejoining her husband and two older daughters until the end of May.

As she approached the well-wishers grouped around her friend from England, Charlotte felt a wistful sense of being left behind. She thrust this emotion aside as unworthy.

Never mind, she told herself soundlessly, you're already two-thirds of the way there! That made her feel better. She caught Emma's eye and moved forward to congratulate her.

William and Caroline were married right after the Glengarry summer. Charlotte's younger brother had found work as a pharmacist, and had moved to Montreal. Their wedding took place on Tuesday, September 8, in the fashionable, cobblestoned foothills of Mount Royal, at the bride's home on McKay Street.

It was solemnized by Dr. Robert Burns, pastor of Côte Street Free Presbyterian Church. Shortly after, the couple left by train for the oceanside village of Huntingdon Sound and a New England honeymoon.

Charlotte's father returned with Charlotte and David to the house in Côte des Neiges. He had a few hours to spend on a visit before leaving that evening for the West. Joseph had won a contract to build sixty-four miles of railway track between Pembina, North Dakota, and St. Boniface, Manitoba. He explained to David that, while the Pembina Branch was not important in itself, it was the supply line that would enable construction to start on the Canadian Pacific westwards.

While the two men talked, Charlotte brewed and served tea. Her father's enthusiasm was contagious. She was reminded of the day he had returned after building the Buffalo, Brantford and Goderich Railway. She had been twelve then; Mary Anne was fourteen. He had come home to The Corners with a quarter of a million dollars stuffed into a carpet bag and a barrel of fine bone china for his daughters. It was from the oblong teapot to this service, with its delicately rendered Oriental birds and flowers, double-banded with gold leaf on ivory white, that Charlotte now poured.

The contract and the trip west by her father were exciting. Equally so was the expectation that her friend Dr. Hingston was soon to be elected mayor of Montreal. Although he was not seeking office and refused to campaign, Hôtel Dieu's chief surgeon was expected to win with a sweep. His name had been put up in the hope that a physician-mayor might bring better health measures to a city too often wracked with contagious disease.

The beginning of Charlotte's third and final session in Philadelphia coincided with a start on the building of the world's first medical school for women. On the first day of October, the cornerstone was laid on College Avenue, right next to Woman's Hospital. It was scheduled to be finished in time for Charlotte and her classmates to be the first graduates. Their final hurdle was the choice of subject for their graduation thesis. It had to be submitted before the last week in January. Since it represented a major addition to their regular studies, most of the students had begun work on theirs immediately after the start of the session.

"How are you doing on your thesis?" Jennie asked Charlotte in mid-October, as they were leaving the lecture hall.

"I'm just about ready to start writing," replied Charlotte. She glanced around her. "Anyone else?"

"Not nearly yet!" said Emily Tefft.

"It's not something you can rush," said Jennie. "So much depends on how well it's researched and written."

Charlotte had an advantage over her classmates. She had chosen her subject and begun researching it at her leisure shortly after her aborted first year.

Early in December, Charlotte sat down one evening at the table in her bedroom and prepared to start writing. She was not concerned with her presentation. She had arranged to have it copied professionally. She studied her notes, then began the first of thirty-six pages. She wrote in a firm scrawl, slowing now and then to form her words more precisely, her thoughts sometimes running away with her fingers: "The subject about to be considered is one of frequent occurrence. The number of mothers passing through the childbearing epoch without aborting once or more is small."

Spontaneous abortion had special significance for Charlotte. She had a history of problem pregnancies, including miscarriage and premature birth. She had also known for almost a month that she was again with child.

"I see no cause for concern," Dr. Cleveland said, after she examined her. "Don't over-exert yourself, and get as much rest as you can. Go to bed early. Get up early. Do your studies from sunup to sundown. Don't stay up half the night!"

"How did you know?" Charlotte asked sheepishly.

"You forget that I, too, was a medical student," Dr. Cleveland replied drily. "Have you written your husband?"

"No, I felt it would only worry him. Besides, he might think I should put off my studies another year. I couldn't do that. Not again."

Dr. Cleveland nodded understandingly. She knew how difficult it had been for Charlotte to repeat her first year and suspend her studies for yet another.

"Well, you're probably right," said Dr. Cleveland. "Just be sure to take good care of yourself."

The new building was completed in time for Commencement. Invitations printed on tinted note paper requested that guests attend at twelve o'clock noon on Thursday, March 11. They were invited to remain afterwards for a reception and an escorted tour of the new facilities.

As one of the school's earliest and staunchest supporters, Sarah Hale was among those present. So were family members and close friends of all the graduates who did not live too far from Philadelphia. Jennie Trout's husband, Edward, had taken time off as publisher of *The Monetary Times* to come down from Toronto. Charlotte had written David in February with the news that he was to be a father again in May. They had discussed in an exchange of letters his coming to her graduation. In the end they had agreed it was too busy a time at Whitehead and Ross and too long a trip from Montreal to Philadelphia.

Now Charlotte was joking with some of her classmates that it had taken her ten years to graduate. "Five years from the day I decided I wanted to be a doctor," she said. "Five more after I was accepted by Woman's Medical!"

David walked to her from across the hall, hands outstretched before he reached her. Charlotte moved apart from the others. Her surprise at seeing him gave way to her great pleasure that he had come. He took both her hands in his.

"Is it Dr. Charlotte Ross, then?" David said. The pride in his voice was unmistakable.

CHAPTER EIGHT

Montreal, Spring, 1875

*T*HE HOUSE AT 895 Ontario Street suited Charlotte perfectly as a home for her family and an office from which she could practise medicine. It was a good address, on the same street as three other physicians, and the Faculty of Medicine of the University of Bishop's College. It was also close to downtown shopping and the city's two hospitals – Hôtel Dieu, and the Royal Victoria.

The house itself was red brick with shuttered windows over grey stone sills. An attic room with dormer, the children's favourite, looked two storeys down on a small entry porch and a lawn fenced by ornamental wrought iron. From the moment she and David had first seen it, Charlotte had known it was just right for the decorous sign now being hung in the parlour window. Neatly lettered in white on a black background, it was just large enough to be read from the street.

> *Charlotte Ross MD*
> *Physician and Accoucheur*
> *Hours: 11 a.m. to 4 p.m.*

Charlotte was standing on the front lawn. The young woman she had hired as housegirl was standing on a chair in the parlour, holding up the sign to the window. "A little higher and to the left!" Charlotte called out. She realized as she spoke that Judith could not hear her. She gestured. Judith raised the sign an inch or so, at the same time moving it slightly to one side. Charlotte vigorously nodded her approval.

"Well now, that looks nice enough." The woman at Charlotte's shoulder was Caroline Kuetzing, a widow, who lived next door. Charlotte had noticed that she spent most of her day on a front-porch rocker, keeping an eye on the street.

"Physician I understand," said Mrs. Kuetzing. "The French word I can't even pronounce."

"*Accoucheur,*" Charlotte obliged. "It means someone who delivers babies."

"Ah," said Mrs. Kuetzing. She gave Charlotte a long look. "Are you really a doctor?"

"I graduated just last month," said Charlotte.

Mrs. Kuetzing considered this. "I never met a lady doctor before," she said.

Charlotte had been pleased to find Judith. A farm girl from the Eastern Townships, she came from a large family and was fond of children. She was almost as strong as a man, and knew her way around a stable. Since David was away so frequently, this was important.

Charlotte had decided to call on the Quebec College of Physicians and Surgeons on the same day that she placed her sign in her window. She asked Judith to hitch up the horse and buggy. In just a few minutes the housegirl brought it around to the front of the house from the stable out back.

Charlotte had had her hair done. Nothing frivolous, of course. Just combed straight back and drawn to a bun at the nape of her neck. She had chosen to wear the full black skirt, white shirtwaist and high-button shoes that she had worn as a student in Philadelphia. For the street she had added black kid gloves and a matching straw cloche. There was a spring chill in the air. She draped a black wool cape over her shoulders.

The College of Physicians and Surgeons had its offices on St. Catherine Street. Charlotte had written the president for an appointment. Immediately on arrival, she was shown into Dr. Robert Russell's office. He sat behind a cleared desk. Another gentleman occupied a chair to one side. Charlotte entered the room to the soundless echoes of a conversation abruptly ended.

"Mrs. Ross," said Dr. Russell, rising.

Charlotte smiled slightly at his choice of salutation. She extended her hand. "Dr. Russell."

He gestured towards his colleague. "This is Dr. Marion. Dr. Marion has his practice less than three blocks from you, on Ontario Street."

"Mrs. Ross," Dr. Marion said curtly.

"Dr. Ross," said Charlotte. "It is Dr. Ross, gentlemen. As I noted in my letter, I am a recent graduate of Woman's Medical College of Pennsylvania."

The two men exchanged a quick look.

"I wish to be admitted to the Quebec College."

"That presents a problem," Dr. Russell said smoothly. "Our bylaws don't allow for membership by a female."

"I would like to know the reason," said Charlotte.

Dr. Russell replied with deliberation. "In mind, emotions and physical makeup, a woman is not suited to the practice of medicine. In matters of morals and modesty, a lady certainly isn't."

"I disagree."

Dr. Russell shrugged. "As you wish. If you practise without being licensed by the College, you will do so illegally. This is punishable by a considerable fine, not just once but as often as necessary." Dr. Russell effected profound regret. "As well, and you force me to say this, dear lady, if you persisted you could face a term in jail. A woman in your position could hardly suffer this lightly."

"I have asked to be recognized by the College and been refused. I had little hope it might be otherwise." Charlotte got to her feet. "I wished simply to make it a matter of record."

Dr. Russell was conciliatory. "Go home and have your baby, Mrs. Ross. No doubt your medical training will equip you better to care for your family."

"As well as a woman," Charlotte said crisply, "I am a qualified doctor." She turned and walked to the door. She waited until Dr. Russell hastened from behind his desk to see her out.

"With or without your approval," Charlotte said, "I intend to practice my profession."

Dr. Russell closed the door behind her. He walked back to his desk and sat down.

Dr. Marion shook his head. "That woman will be trouble."

"Trouble?" Dr. Russell repeated. "You forget it is the College that decides who practises in Quebec. If necessary we can give Mrs. Ross a great deal more trouble than she bargained for."

Charlotte left the College's offices in a good frame of mind. The meeting had gone exactly as she thought it would. She hummed softly to herself as she slipped the reins from the hitching post outside the building and got back into her buggy. She set off for Bonsecours Market to keep the second of the two appointments she had made for that day.

Dr. Hingston had someone with him when Charlotte arrived. She had to wait only briefly in the anteroom outside his office before the mayor saw his earlier visitor out. He gave Charlotte a warm smile. It was their first meeting since her return from Philadelphia.

"Dr. Ross!" he exclaimed over a courtly bow. "Welcome and congratulations!" He turned to his secretary. "Thomas, I do not wish to be disturbed." Then again to Charlotte, "Do please come in."

"It is I who should congratulate you," said Charlotte. "You will be good for the city. Everyone's already applauding your campaign against smallpox."

"Not everyone," Dr. Hingston said wryly. "I've already had two visits from Emery Coderre. He and his supporters are threatening violence if vaccination is made law." He shook his head. "I always considered Coderre a competent doctor. In this matter he is deaf to logic and blind to evidence."

Dr. Hingston brightened. "Enough of the mayor and his problems. What of Dr. Charlotte Ross?"

"I have just come from seeing Dr. Russell. He promised the College would prosecute if I went into practice."

"It has prosecuted in the past, but only against charlatans. Never against a graduate of a recognized medical school." Dr. Hingston was thoughtful. "As mayor of Montreal I am also chief magistrate. I will ask Chief Penton to report any action taken against you."

"I am under your protection then?"

"Of course."

Charlotte nodded. They both knew it was the assurance she needed for her to practise in Montreal.

"I have become engaged," said Dr. Hingston.

"To Margaret Josephine?"

"Yes. She and her sisters are moving to Toronto soon with their father. He has been appointed lieutenant governor of Ontario. We'll be married there in September."

"I'm sure you'll be very happy," said Charlotte. "As my dear friend, I wish that for you. And for Margaret Josephine."

On a Tuesday morning in mid-May, Charlotte was seated at her desk in the room she had fitted out as her office. David had left the previous day for a week-long sales trip through the Eastern Townships. Charlotte had seen her three older daughters off to school. Carrie was playing in the fenced backyard while Judith kept an eye of her from the kitchen window. Charlotte was consulting one of her medical-school textbooks, Parrish's *Practical Pharmacy,* about a prescription compound William had asked about.

Her first labour pain had come while she was still in bed. It had begun imperceptibly enough in the small of her back, gently nudging her out of a sound sleep. It's too soon, she thought, changing to a more comfortable position. But as she slowly came awake she asked herself, Isn't it always? After a few moments the pain had subsided. She sighed and smiled at the ceiling, gently clasping her hands on the rounded bedclothes. "God bless you," she said aloud. "You've shown more patience than your sisters!"

Now in her office she felt another spasm and placed a hand on her belly, feeling for contractions. She glanced at the clock on the mantel board. Then she went back to the book she was reading. When the next spasm came she saw that just under fifteen minutes had passed. She pushed the book away from her. She could hear Judith moving about in the kitchen. Charlotte got up and walked to the hallway.

"Judith."

The housegirl poked her head out the kitchen doorway.

"You had better go for the doctor."

Judith smiled broadly and fumbled for her apron strings. "Yes, ma'am!"

The baby was born just past midday. It was a boy.

Judith plumped the pillows, beaming over Charlotte and the sleeping infant she held at her breast. "Should I bring the children now?"

Charlotte nodded. She had not had an easy time. She had never been blessed with uncomplicated pregnancies and simple births. When hers did not end in miscarriage, they invariably were premature and difficult. This time, though, she felt a special sense of satisfaction. It was for David. She had finally given her husband a son. Judith paused at the bedroom door. "Mr. Ross will be so proud," she said. "Have you picked a name yet?"

Charlotte had talked this over with David. He had left the choice to her.

"Hales," she said. "Hales Hingston Ross."

Charlotte was the only woman among Montreal's 142 practising physicians and surgeons. Her practice grew quickly. Her patients were women and children, all drawn by the sign in her parlour window or referrals by friends and neighbours. Maureen Lesage had heard of Charlotte through a friend. She was an Irish woman, born and brought up in Griffintown, who had married a French Canadian. She and her husband, Henri, had five children, the youngest four years old. They lived just a few blocks from Ontario Street, on Chenneville. Charlotte had been treating the older brother and three sisters for fairly severe cases of influenza. It had been passed from one child to the other over the previous few weeks. Mrs. Lesage was standing in wait for Charlotte when she came to the door.

"Robert's fever seems worse!" She took a quick step back, hoping to hasten Charlotte's entry. "I bathed him with cold towels like you told me to. It hasn't helped."

Charlotte frowned. "His fever should have broken by now." It had been four days since the young Lesage boy had begun showing the same 'flu symptoms as his brother and sisters. Head and backaches. Alternately shivering from chills and perspiring from fever.

"He has a small rash on his face," said his mother.

Charlotte looked at her sharply. "Has he been vomiting?"

"Yes. Last night and again early this morning."

Charlotte started up the stairs. Symptoms just like those of influenza, she thought. No way to diagnose the disease accurately until the rash appears. Then it comes out on the forehead, the scalp, wrists and feet. She swept down the hall to the boy's bedroom. She knew what to look for and found it, just as she feared she would. Robert was lying between damp bedclothes. He had the hot look of fever in his eyes. A cluster of bright red spots was beginning to rise on his forehead. Soon they would fill with clear fluid, putrefy and erupt. Charlotte walked to him. She set her black leather medical bag down on a bedside table. "Hello, Robert."

"Hello." The voice came small and weak. Charlotte's heart went out to the boy with the hand she gently placed on his forehead. She felt his mother's presence behind her.

"Your son has smallpox."

The woman's knuckles flew to her lips. "Good God in heaven!"

Charlotte straightened. She pulled the pins from her shirtwaist cuffs and pushed back her sleeves. She gestured towards the window. "Take down the curtains." She stooped and began rolling up the carpet. "Smallpox is very contagious. I don't want anyone but us coming into this room. Understand?"

They stored the curtains and rug in the basement. "We'll need linens," Charlotte said. "Lots of them."

While Mrs. Lesage tore these into wash and drying cloths, Charlotte mixed a strong solution of carbolic acid and water. A full sheet was soaked, wrung out and hung over the entrance to the sickroom. Charlotte poured more of the antiseptic solution into the chamber pot and covered it with a soaked square of linen. She filled the ironstone pitcher and basin on the bedroom bureau and stacked cloths beside them.

"Use these to wipe his nose and mouth. Then burn them in the stove. Wash before you leave the room. Leave the wash cloths to soak, and burn the cloths you use for towels." Charlotte glanced around the room. "Now we need two pails of hot water – one with shaved soap and lye, the other clear, I want this room scrubbed clean every morning. Use a paring knife at the baseboards. I'll show you how."

Robert's mother was hard put to keep up with Charlotte. She did not mind. She had growing confidence in this compact woman with the quick, positive manner who delivered instructions with such crisp authority.

Charlotte got back home in late afternoon. The sounds of her children playing in the backyard came to her through the screen door in the kitchen. She heard Judith asking them to please be a little more quiet because their mother couldn't work with all that racket going on. The sounds died down. They started up again louder than ever at the sharp slap of the spring-shut screen door as Judith returned to the kitchen. Charlotte smiled at her mutter of goodnatured resignation over the rattle of dishes. A few moments later, Judith entered with a tray.

"I brought you a nice hot cup of tea and some sugar cookies I just baked," she said. "I asked the children not to be so noisy."

Charlotte smiled. "I heard."

"It didn't help much."

"It doesn't matter. Usually when children are having fun they're healthy. That's what counts."

Early the next morning, Charlotte began a daily routine in her treatment of the Lesage boy. His mother spent most of every night at his bedside. Shortly after Charlotte arrived, she lay down and napped until Charlotte was finished. After the first few days, Charlotte realized that the woman was not physically able to maintain indefinitely her night-long vigil over her son, care for the rest of her family and scrub down the sickroom daily.

Charlotte first looked in on Robert. When she came back downstairs, his mother was doing up the breakfast dishes. She pulled her cuff pins and began rolling up the sleeves of her shirtwaist. "Where do you keep the wash buckets?"

Mrs. Lesage gestured with her dishcloth towards a kitchen closet. "In there." She coloured, realizing why Charlotte had asked. "I'm sorry. I haven't had time yet to do Robert's room."

Charlotte walked to the closet and hauled out the two buckets. "You're not going to. I am."

"Please! I can't let you do that!"

"Hush!" Charlotte dropped the scrub brush into one of the buckets. "There's one member of this family sick already. I don't want another."

She took a tin of lye and a bottle of carbolic acid from her medical bag. "When you' re done there I want you to get some sleep."

Mrs. Lesage capitulated. "It's been a long night," she admitted.

"The first of many," said Charlotte. "We've got three more weeks of this."

Upstairs, Charlotte drew aside the sheet at the doorway to Robert's room and went to his bedside. "How are you feeling, Robert?"

The boy did not reply. He looked up at her through eyes as hot and hooded-grey as ashen embers. She leaned closer and he frowned, weakly reaching out to her. His fingers touched and lingered on the coolness of her cheek. Charlotte took his hand in hers and pressed it to her lips.

"With God's help," she whispered.

She filled the basin by his bed with a mild solution of carbolic acid and warm water. She gently bathed him. Then she dried and lightly dusted him with boric powder. She changed his nightshirt and bedclothes, which were sweaty and wrinkled. Satisfied that he was comfortable, she picked up the wash buckets and carried them to the far end of the room. She took the scrub brush in one hand, hitched up her skirts with the other, and knelt to work.

In the days that followed, Charlotte arrived early at the Lesages' and stayed late. She prepared bags of chipped ice for the boy's fevers, and held him in her arms when he shook from cold. She gave him antiseptic bedbaths daily, followed by dustings with boric powder for the rash that became blisters, festered like boils, then burst on the twelfth day and scabbed. For long periods she sat at his bedside, gently holding the ice bag in place when the fever made him fitful. Sometimes she just sat with her hand on his forehead, seeking to touch him with the wordless prayer that came so straight from her heart that it left her lips unmoved.

Maureen Lesage was wakened by low voices, punctuated by an oddly piercing sound. She had lain down when Charlotte came, and had dropped off to sleep. The odd noise was repeated over and over, sometimes trailing off in a dry wheeze. The sounds were coming from her son's room. She got up and hurried down the hall.

Charlotte was perched on the edge of the bed, lips puckered, blowing soundlessly. Robert was sitting up, frowning concentration as he tried to set his lips in precisely the same way.

Charlotte turned and faced the boy's mother. "We are learning how to whistle," she said.

It was later that week, just after Charlotte's children had left for school, that she found Judith nudging in through the front door with a pail of soapy water in one hand and a wet cloth in the other. Charlotte was on her way downstairs. "You're certainly getting an early start on your housework." She paused on a stair. Judith looked flustered, like Bella had a week or so earlier when Charlotte had surprised her in her office, leafing through Gray's *Anatomy*. "Is something wrong, Judith?"

"No, ma'am." Judith averted her eyes as she pushed the door shut with her shoulder and started down the hall to the kitchen.

"Judith."

"Ma'am?"

"It seems to me you washed down the front entrance just yesterday."

Judith kept her eyes from Charlotte's. "Someone's been writing on the front door."

"What kind of writing?" Charlotte descended the last few steps to the stairwell and walked to the door. "Is this the first time?"

"No, ma'am."

"You should have told me, Judith."

Charlotte suppressed a smile. Standing in the hallway with her wash cloth and pail and good intentions, the simple country girl looked as wretched as a scarecrow in winter. "I'm sure you thought to be considerate," Charlotte said. "But if it happens again, I want you to tell me."

"Yes, ma'am!" With a look of relief, Judith disappeared into the kitchen.

Charlotte opened the door and stepped outside. There was

126

no trace of the offending words. Charlotte could imagine what they had been – the same crude sort that Jennie Trout and Emily Stowe's classmates had written on the walls of the Toronto School of Medicine. Bishop's College was just two blocks up the street. She decided that if the vulgar act were repeated, she would speak to the dean.

Charlotte was looking forward to an exciting summer. They were celebrating Bella's thirteenth birthday just three days before Dominion Day. Then she and David were leaving for Toronto to meet with her stepmother at the McDonalds'. They planned to visit with Margaret's brother and his family over the weekend, then board the Great Western Railway for Detroit, Chicago and the West. Joseph had invited them to spend a month or so at his construction headquarters, a cluster of tents near St. Boniface on the banks of the Red River.

All three of them were quick to accept. Margaret had complained of having had only brief glimpses of her husband since he had begun work on the Pembina Branch the previous fall. Charlotte had known ever since her talk with David in Clinton six years earlier that he was interested in moving west. She also knew that he had put this interest on hold because of her studies in Philadelphia. "You deserve this chance to see what it's like," she said. "Besides, if we're going to move, I want some idea of what we're getting into!" It amused Charlotte that what she referred to as "western fever" was highly contagious. Epidemic, in fact. Hanna had written, saying that she and Charles were interested in hearing what she thought of the opportunities. William had asked her to find out about pharmacies.

"I can see it now," he said. "First a drugstore or two in Winnipeg. Then a chain across the North-West!"

Charlotte laughed outright. She had always been both amused and charmed, as most people were, by William's runaway enthusiasms.

A week before they were due to leave, Charlotte stepped out of the house into the sweet warmth of late spring melding into early summer. Ordinarily, she would have stopped to savour the bunched amethyst blossoms on the French lilacs that grew by the porch. Today she was too occupied with plans for Bella's birthday and the trip west. As Charlotte descended the steps and walked to the buggy, she noticed a jumble of white on the driver's seat. At first she thought Judith had overlooked something bought that morning at the market. When she realized what it was, Charlotte picked up one of the bones. Her annoyance gave way to disgust at this final indignity to another human being. She went back to the house for a shoe box.

Bishop's College was just a brief trot up the street. When Charlotte had tethered her horse and buggy by the entrance, she took down the shoe box from the driver's seat and tucked it under one arm.

Dr. Aaron David, the dean of the Medical Faculty, was at work at his desk. Since the day was already uncomfortably close, he was seated in his shirtsleeves and waistcoat. He absently called out to enter at Charlotte's knock.

"Dr. David?"

At the sound of her voice, the dean glanced up and quickly got to his feet. He took his suitcoat from a clothes tree by his desk and put it on. "I'm sorry," he said. "I wasn't expecting anyone."

Charlotte dismissed his apology with a smile. "It's quite warm for June."

"And humid."

Charlotte nodded. She found that Montreal could be uncomfortably close in summer, although not usually this early. Dr. David placed a chair in front of his desk. "Do please be seated, Mrs. . . . ?"

"Dr. Charlotte Ross."

The dean acknowledged the introduction with a nod. As he walked back behind his desk, Charlotte assessed his manner. She thought it to be guardedly curious. Obviously he had heard of her. Quite possibly, walking or riding along Ontario Street to Bishop's, he had seen the sign in her parlour window. Almost certainly she had been discussed by his faculty colleagues and students. Friend or foe? Charlotte idly wondered which. She remained standing and placed the shoe box on the dean's desk. "I believe these belong here at Bishop's."

Dr. David lifted the lid of the box and frowned at its contents. "I found them on the seat of my buggy."

"I see."

"A mindless prank," said Charlotte.

"I agree."

"There have been other, more personally offensive incidents. Vulgarities scribbled on the door to my home. I believe some of your students may be responsible."

Dr. David's frown deepened. "I was not aware."

"I felt certain you weren't."

The dean placed the lid back on the box. "As regrettable as the circumstances are that brought you here, Dr. Ross, they do give us an opportunity to talk."

"Please do."

"You must realize you are bound to encounter a great deal of prejudice. I am aware of your situation. You have been denied admission to the Quebec College. You have chosen to practise, regardless."

"I was refused because I am a woman. I don't accept that as a valid reason."

Dr. David shrugged. "That's a matter for you, your conscience and possibly the courts to decide. Like most of my colleagues, I do not approve of ladies in medicine. In some departments, such as midwifery, perhaps. In most others, surgery for instance, it is generally felt that women lack the required nerve."

"You are entitled to your view," said Charlotte. "As you say, it is not an uncommon one."

"To be sure." Seeing that Charlotte was about to leave, the dean got up. "Whatever one's personal convictions," he said, gesturing towards the shoe box, "this sort of mindless prank, as you so charitably call it, is reprehensible. Even more so is the other form of harassment to which you were subjected. I will speak to my students. You may rest assured there will be no further incidents."

Charlotte turned to go.

"Dr. Ross."

"Yes?"

"I sympathize with your problem. I was the first Jew to graduate and practise medicine in this country. I am no stranger to prejudice."

Charlotte studied him for a moment. "Then you should know it has many disguises," she said.

Dr. David thought about Charlotte's parting remark as he took off his suitcoat and replaced it on its hanger. At the same time, he was reminded of the comment made by Dr. Francis Campbell, secretary-treasurer of the Faculty of Medicine, whenever the subject of women doctors came up. "Imagine a critically ill patient," Dr. Campbell would say, "waiting for half an hour while the medical lady fixes her bonnet, or adjusts her bustle!" The remark always brought a ripple of amusement from his audience. As often as he had heard it, Dr. David chuckled at this imagined absurdity.

CHAPTER ❦ NINE

St. Boniface, Summer, 1875

*T*HE HOT AND HUMID DAYS of June that had begun Charlotte's summer in Montreal followed her out west. With David and her stepmother, she was among forty-five passengers to leave Moorhead, Minnesota, aboard a paddle-wheeler called the SS Selkirk.

Even on the river, they found it too close to get much sleep their first night out and again on the second. On the third day, before the first call to breakfast in the dining lounge, they met on the passenger deck to catch whatever breeze they could. The boat was negotiating a long bend in the river. Once around, it came upon a small Manitoba settlement off the port bow. The giant paddlewheel in the stern was reduced to a lazy turning. Standing on the deck beneath the wheelhouse and the boat's two tall smokestacks, they watched as the captain eased towards the dock at Scratching River.

The SS Selkirk was one of seven mixed passenger and freight boats that plied the Red as far north as Winnipeg and St. Boniface. The two towns faced each other across the river. While the crew unloaded boxes and sacks of freight from the main deck, David escorted Charlotte and Margaret on a walk along the riverbank. At each step a pale green cloud of grasshoppers sprang from underfoot. Charlotte had known summers back east when people talked about infestations of grasshoppers. She had never seen anything like this. She found that if the three of them stood still and listened, they could hear the eerie murmur of them eating.

The SS Selkirk came in sight of Winnipeg and St. Boniface with a series of short, hoarse hurrahs on its steamwhistle. Among the dockside crowd that turned out to meet it was Charlotte's father. Margaret was the first to see and call out to her husband. She leaned into the deckrail, plucking a lace handkerchief from the wristband of her dress and waving it until she caught his eye. Joseph smiled broadly, returning the wave and doffing his hat to his wife and daughter. He was standing with one of his foremen. A group of teamsters lounged nearby, waiting with their wagons to cart supplies off to camp. While David and the foreman loaded their luggage onto one of the wagons, Joseph spoke with Charlotte and Margaret.

"Did you have a good trip out?"

"Quite comfortable," said his wife, "except for the heat." Her handkerchief fluttered to her forehead. "I suppose it's been no better here."

"The same," said Joseph. "Intolerable."

"At our last stop we went ashore," said Charlotte. "Is there always such a plague of grasshoppers?"

Her father shook his head. "They've been unusually bad this summer and last. They're eating everything in sight. The Hudson's Bay Company store has barricaded itself behind packing cases topped with tin. It's too high for them to jump and too slippery to climb. When they grow wings we'll be well rid of them!"

Joseph's Pembina Branch headquarters and base camp was just a short wagon ride south along the riverbank from St. Boniface. Charlotte and David shared the driver's seat with a young teamster, their trunk and smaller pieces of luggage bouncing around with the boxes and sacks of provisions he had loaded in back. Joseph and Margaret sat up front in the lead wagon with the foreman at the reins. Both women rode most of the way with one gloved hand on their wide-brimmed straw hats. The other gripped the handrail by their sides. In the few words exchanged over the rattle and lurch of the wagon, Charlotte and David's driver said he was a homesteader whose crops had been wiped out for the second year by grasshoppers. Charlotte thought he took this remarkably well, shrugging it off as just one of the hardships of farming in the West. He was working for Mr. Whitehead as a teamster to keep his homestead and his family fed until they had a good harvest. His eyes, as clear and blue as the prairie sky, were confident. "Next year," he said.

As relieved as Charlotte and her stepmother were to reach the campsite, it contrasted badly with the elegant lounges and comfortable staterooms of the paddlewheeler. Charlotte and David's tent was outfitted with canvas cots, a chair, a washstand with a tin water jug and basin, a chamber pot and a coal-oil lantern that hung from the centre pole. Joseph and Margaret's tent was the same, with the addition of a second chair and a small table where Joseph did his paperwork. A third tent was set up with an old oak dining table, four chairs and a bedroom bureau that served as a sideboard.

There were grasshoppers everywhere. It was even worse than at Scratching River. Joseph warned them that whatever was not safely stored in their trunk would be eaten. After a walk around the campsite, Charlotte and David joined Joseph and Margaret for afternoon tea in the dining tent. Charlotte left her straw hat lying on her cot. She returned to find that its brim had been eaten ragged.

"I told you the little beggars would eat anything," Joseph teased her at dinner.

Charlotte was not amused. "I didn't realize you meant just *anything*!" she said. "I bought that hat at Henry Morgan's just before we left!"

"Apart from that," Joseph addressed his wife, "how do you like your first taste of the West?"

Margaret wrinkled her nose. "It's alive with those destructive pests. It's hot. And it's uncomfortable. I can't for the life of me imagine why anyone would choose to live here."

"Opportunity," said Joseph. "Just a few years ago, William Luxton came out from the East to teach school." He reached for *The Daily Free Press* he had put down when the cook-tent boy had brought their dinner trays. "Now he's a member of the Manitoba Legislative Assembly, and he and his partner own the West's first daily newspaper." He opened it to an inside page. "He

136

has an amusing view of how hot it is," he said, reading aloud. "'Parasols, fans, linen coats, melted paper collars, laziness, lemonade, peeled noses, perspiration and soda water were today's amusements. Hot was no name for it.'"

The droll description made Charlotte smile. "I can see why an ambitious man would find the West attractive." She was thinking of both David and the young homesteader who had driven them to the campsite. His spirit had impressed her. He had been so confident of good crops to come and his own and his family's future.

"It's such a vast and empty place," said her stepmother. "So much needs doing!"

"By those who don't mind hard work," said David.

"Exactly," said Joseph. "You have no idea. Building the railway – everything is so much more difficult than back east. There's a shortage of skilled workers. We've poor roads, or none at all. Freighting has to be done by riverboat and oxcart." He shook his head.

"But outweighing all of that?" David prompted.

Joseph grinned at his son-in-law. "At least a hundred ways to make your fortune."

The next morning, Charlotte and Margaret crossed over to Winnipeg by cable ferry. When it docked they picked their way past bales and boxes to where the freight teamsters and top-hatted liverymen stood waiting with their oxcarts and carriages. The sun was not yet high enough in the sky to make walking too much effort. They asked directions to Main Street from one of the drivers. Amid the clatter of passing buggies, work crews and horse-drawn scrapers, Charlotte and Margaret walked carefully. They hitched up their skirts to step nimbly past workmen laying storm pipe. They stopped to stare at a stuffed grasshopper in a shop window. A card labelled it the "Boss 'Hopper – 96 pounds." Charlotte rolled her eyes at Margaret and they both laughed, moving on up the street. It was not much further to the Grand Canada Hotel, where they had arranged to have luncheon with Joseph and David. Later they planned to do the shops, including the pharmacy count for William.

Joseph and David had just come from a meeting with the man who ran the freight line. With his partner, James McKay owned several hundred oxcarts. A onetime Hudson's Bay Company scout and buffalo hunter, he was also Manitoba's Minister of Agriculture.

"McKay's a half-breed," Joseph said over luncheon. "He's a huge man. I'd say well over three hundred pounds. His wife, Margaret, is cast from the same mould. They drive a two-horse carriage custom-built to carry their weight."

"You can't be serious," said Margaret.

"As God's my witness!" said Joseph. "They're well off. They live in a mansion called Deer Lodge just west of town, on the Portage la Prairie Road. It's said to have the best wine cellar in the West."

"Do they have any children?" asked Charlotte.

"Three of their own and an adopted daughter – a full-blooded

Sioux Indian. About ten years ago, the child and her mother arrived hungry at the McKays' door. James and Margaret took them in. They gave the woman the Christian name Harriett and the girl Augusta."

"The McKays must be good people," said Margaret. "That was an unusual thing to do, even out here."

Charlotte and her stepmother spent most of their stay in and around camp, or had one of the men drive them into St. Boniface. Charlotte was interested in the men working on the Pembina Branch and the care provided those who were injured. She and Margaret stopped by St. Boniface Hospital, which was just a log cabin with four beds, none of them occupied. The hospital was run by a French-speaking member of the Sisters of Charity, popularly known, from the colour of their habit, as the Grey Nuns; she was not long out from Montreal. The nun was surprised when Charlotte said she was a doctor. She was even more surprised when Charlotte told her that she was in general practice there. The sister had assumed she was a missionary. She was familiar with Hôtel Dieu and yes, of course, the exceptional work of its chief surgeon, but she had never met Dr. Hingston personally.

The nun told Charlotte that most of their accidents were axe cuts or related to millwork and horse-drawn machinery. She said the most common diseases were *typhoïde, petite vérole* and *phtisie.* Charlotte translated these for Margaret as typhoid fever, smallpox and consumption. While Charlotte was still speaking to her stepmother, the sister frowned and added a fourth. *"Alcool."* With a resigned Gallic shrug she said that perhaps none of the preceding three was as big a problem as alcohol.

The evening before their departure, Charlotte was helping her stepmother clear the dishes in the dining tent. Joseph had gone to speak with his foreman of teamsters about the next day's work. David had gone with him. Margaret picked up a copy of *The Daily Free Press* that her husband had left behind on the sideboard. It was folded open at the editorial page.

"This will interest you," she said. "It's called 'Women as Physicians.'"

"What does it say?"

"They've decided to let women practise medicine in England."

Charlotte put down some plates and took the newspaper from Margaret.

A few months earlier, Jennie Trout had met the requirements of the College of Physicians and Surgeons and had become the first woman licensed to practise medicine in Canada. While in fact this meant only Ontario, it was the first step. Now her old friend and classmate Emma Palmer could be licensed in England. Charlotte read William Luxton's editorial comment: "Great Britain is thus to have female doctors who, if they confine themselves to treating their own sex, will do a great deal of good service."

The statement brought a smile to Charlotte's face. She

wondered what Emma would have said about anything so charitably patronizing.

Charlotte and David came away from Manitoba impressed with much of what they had seen and heard. Charlotte knew that her husband was intrigued by the challenge of the West. She was also aware that he was disenchanted with his role as a drummer for Whitehead and Ross. The man she had married liked to work with his hands and have his own door to come home to when the work was done. David had once managed a sawmill for Charlotte's father. It was at a small settlement called Bandon, not far from Clinton, on the banks of the Maitland River. In those early years of their marriage, Charlotte thought she had never seen her husband happier.

During their visit to St. Boniface, Joseph had told them that he was confident of being awarded two more railway-construction contracts. One was an extension of the Pembina Branch – twenty-two miles of track northeast from St. Boniface to Selkirk. Eventually, he said, this stretch would bring the railway into Winnipeg.

The second was called Contract 15. It was over thirty-seven miles of forest and rock, rivers and muskeg, from Rat Portage, on Lake of the Woods, to Cross Lake, on the Canadian Pacific's main line west.

Joseph had said that he was going to need vast quantities of railway ties, timbers for trestles and dressed lumber for camp buildings. He wanted David to set up and run the mill. He was offering Charles the job of his own second-in-command and general troubleshooter.

Charlotte and David had talked it over on the long trip by riverboat and railway back through the United States to the border crossing at Detroit and Windsor. She did not doubt that both her husband and her older brother would accept Joseph's offer. She was just as certain that what she had found out about opportunities for pharmacists would convince William that his future, too, was in the West.

During Charlotte and David's absence there had been anti-vaccination riots in Montreal. A small but fanatic medical faction led by Dr. Coderre was campaigning publicly that vaccination did not immunize against smallpox. They claimed, instead, that it infected those vaccinated with the disease. In mid-August a mob had stoned City Hall and set fire to the St. Catherine Street office of Dr. A.B. Larocque, the medical health officer.

Open and violent opposition to Dr. Hingston's medical and civic authority spilled over into Charlotte's practice. Under his protection as mayor and chief magistrate, she had managed to force entry into the traditional men's club of Quebec medicine. Quite apart from the usual prejudice against women, the growing success of her practice was costing some Montreal doctors money. Charlotte knew that this – not just her being a women – was ultimately what they would find intolerable.

"You go right in."

Charlotte was checking a patient's file in her office when she heard Judith's voice from the entry hall. She had been so engrossed in the file that she was not aware that someone had entered. She looked up as Judith showed in a young woman. The girl made a slight curtsy. "I'm Mrs. Johnson's housegirl, ma'am." She spoke breathlessly. There were high spots on her cheeks. "Mrs. Johnson thinks her baby's due. She wants you to come."

Charlotte turned to Judith, who was standing in the doorway. "Bring 'round the buggy." Judith disappeared, and Charlotte took her visitor by the elbow. "Sit down and rest a moment."

Mrs. Johnson's housegirl sat gratefully. "I came as fast as I could."

Charlotte was checking the contents of her medical bag. She smiled at the young woman. "I'm sure you did."

"I had to leave my rig and run the last part. The street's blocked."

Charlotte snapped shut her bag. "Blocked? How?"

"There's a hackney carriage parked at each end. I tried both ways, but they wouldn't let me through."

Charlotte frowned. "Did anyone tell you why?"

"No, ma'am. They just asked me where I was going. When I told them Dr. Ross's, they told me no. They said to turn and go back home."

Charlotte considered this while she drew on her gloves. She decided that the most plausible explanation was almost, but not quite, too outrageous. She heard Judith draw up in front with the buggy and picked up her bag. "Come along."

Charlotte waited on the porch for the housegirl to catch up with her. To the right, down past Mrs. Kuetzing's house, was Bleury Street. To the left was Balmoral. Charlotte saw that a carriage blocked Ontario Street at both intersections. At Balmoral, a hackney man lolled by his horse's head, one hand loosely holding the bridle. At Bleury, the driver sat in the carriage, hunched over his reins. Judith sensed something was wrong. As she stepped down from the buggy she glanced up and down the street. "What's this about?"

Charlotte took her place in the driver's seat. "We'll soon see."

Judith was instantly protective. "Do you want me to go with you?"

Charlotte shook her head. "You stay here with the children. If the Johnson baby is premature, I could be gone a while."

"Well, if you're sure," Judith said uncertainly.

"I'm sure."

Charlotte waited for Mrs. Johnson's housegirl to take the seat beside her. She lightly slapped the reins across her horse's back and moved up the street towards Balmoral. The hackney man standing by his carriage straightened, watching their approach. When they were close enough for him to recognize the housegirl he had turned back earlier, he planted his feet apart and took a firm hold on his horse's bridle. Charlotte drew up a short piece before the intersection.

"Make way!" she called out.

The man shook his head. "Not today, missy."

Charlotte ignored his impudence. "I am Dr. Ross. I am on my

way to minister to an expectant mother."

"I well know who you are. You'll not be seeing any expectant mothers today. Or tomorrow, either."

"By whose order?"

The hackney man shrugged.

Charlotte studied him for a moment. The man was a layabout, as common to the streets of lower Montreal as cobblestones, as ready for this kind of work as for hacking. She decided to waste no further words on him. She called out, "Gee-haw!" and tugged on the right rein. The horse and buggy turned tightly about in the street and started back at a walk the way it had come.

"You'll get no further that end!" the man shouted after her.

Charlotte was furious. It made no difference that she had already decided to close her Montreal practice. She was determined that no one, especially by so brutish an action, was going to do it for her. She was opposite her house. She drew up and turned the buggy again, facing back towards Balmoral. She spoke reassuringly to the girl seated beside her. "Don't be afraid." She took the whip from its box by the seat. "Hold on." She waited for her passenger to grasp the handrail by her side. Charlotte gave a shout. She half-rose, laying the whip across her horse's hindquarters and charging back the way she had come.

The hackney man had slouched again, a slack hand on his horse's bridle. He jerked upright.

Charlotte's father had taught her from childhood how to handle a horse and buggy. She drove well. She knew where she must pull up not to crash into the hackney carriage. "Almost now," she told herself. "Almost, . . . almost . . ."

She saw the hackney man's frightened face as he abruptly shoved on the bridle; saw his horse rear, blowing and snorting, as he crowded it back into the gutter; heard his shouts above the clatter of hooves and wheels.

Charlotte slowed to a stop. She glanced at her young passenger. Mrs. Johnson's housegirl sat ramrod straight, both hands clamped to the handrail. They both looked back and saw the hackney man too busy bringing his horse to hand to care whether they came or went. They started to laugh.

Less than two months later, as October rains dimpled the St. Lawrence, and the trees on Mount Royal became coloured umbrellas, Charlotte and David left Montreal.

CHAPTER ❦ TEN

Clinton, Winter, 1877

*C*HARLOTTE HAD KEPT BUSY over the three months since her return from Montreal. Her stepmother had caught a severe cold in late fall that had lingered on. Her condition had left much of the running of the house to Charlotte, and all the usual preparations for the Christmas-to-hogmanay week.

Charlotte had also made a point of spending as much time as she could with her niece and nephew. Mary Anne's daughter, Josephine, was almost fifteen. William was eleven. Was it really eight years since her sister had died? Charlotte regretted that she had not been able to see as much of the children as she would have liked. Living in Montreal, with only the occasional visit to Clinton, had made this impossible.

It amused her that as big as her father's house was, it had seemed filled to overflowing with children over the past while. She had seen to it that Mary Anne's were frequent guests. Charles, Hanna and their three had moved in from Blyth just before Christmas.

Joseph had been awaiting official word from Ottawa that he had been awarded Contract 15. Confirmation had arrived the first week in January. It had come from the office of Alexander Mackenzie, the Liberal who was now prime minister. Sir John A. Macdonald and his Conservatives had resigned in disgrace over kickbacks revealed by the Canadian Pacific Railway scandal. Within the week, Charlotte's father, her elder brother and her husband had left by rail for the West.

Charlotte was concerned for her stepmother. Margaret had been unable to shake the infection that had begun as a simple cold. She was afraid that it might be developing into something more serious.

Charlotte saw that she was awake and drew up a chair beside her. "Are you feeling any better?"

Margaret's nod did not deceive her. She knew her stepmother to be the selfless kind of woman who seldom had time for personal illness. It had been just over the past few days that Margaret had agreed to rest in bed.

"Here. Let me help you sit up a minute."

Her stepmother's breathing was laboured, uneven. Over her weak protests, Charlotte plumped up the pillows. She undid her stepmother's nightdress and placed her middle finger on her chest. She bent close to listen while she tapped the back of her hand with her other middle finger. The note she heard as she moved her hands across Margaret's chest was not clearly resonant, as it should have been, but flat. Charlotte frowned. She got up and left the room, returning in a few moments with her stethoscope. She held the bell to Margaret's chest. Charlotte caught the faint click of rales, the sound made by moisture in the air sacs of the lungs. She removed the stethoscope, buttoned her stepmother's nightdress, and gently re-arranged the pillows.

"Did you find anything?" Margaret asked.

"Nothing to worry about." Charlotte tucked her in and kissed her forehead. "Nothing a little rest won't help."

She got up and walked to the door. She closed it softly behind her and stood for a moment. Her examination had told her that her stepmother had pneumonia.

Although Charlotte had not gone into practice in Clinton as she had in Montreal, Margaret was not her only patient. Dr. Cole had died two years earlier at fifty-eight. Margaret had described his funeral as the biggest the town had ever seen. There was no doubt that Dr. Cole had been both overworked and charitable, as many of his friends and patients said, but hardly, in Charlotte's opinion, to a fault. Like Dr. Cole, she believed in the upper-class Victorian ethic that privilege brought with it responsibility. As well as a few patients of her own from among friends and neighbours, Charlotte had quietly inherited many of Dr. Cole's less affluent ones.

There was little that she could do for her stepmother. She gave her daily chest and back rubs with alcohol and oil. These and mustard plasters helped to loosen the phlegm that gave her so much discomfort. Mostly they served only to make her condition more tolerable. She had been steadily deteriorating over the previous several days.

Pneumonia was called "the dying man's friend." In terminally ill patients, the fluid that filled the lungs brought on a merciful end. Charlotte was not prepared to accept this for her step-mother. Margaret was an otherwise healthy woman. What concerned Charlotte was the knowledge that pneumonia in someone past middle age often led to kidney or heart failure. Her stepmother was fifty-two.

Margaret's condition grew worse. Old blood from ruptured lung tissues rusted her sputum. From early Wednesday through the day and night into Thursday, Charlotte sat by the low flame of the coal-oil lamp at Margaret's bedside. Cyanosis had set in. Diminished oxygen from her damaged lungs gave a pale blue cast to her complexion. Charlotte held her when she cried out at the sharp pains from her panicked heart.

Just before light, Margaret slept. In her own bedroom, Charlotte agonized over just how temporal her skills were. The diploma that hung on the wall mocked her. Finally, after a long while, she realized that this was not fair – not to her profession, not to herself. The time had simply come when Margaret's life was in God's hands. There was nothing more that she nor anyone else could do but hope and pray for her.

When she heard the housegirl and her husband in the kitchen, Charlotte knew it was seven o'clock. Alex Straiton would soon be starting out for the railway station and telegraph office. She lighted her way downstairs to the writing desk in the parlour. She took out a pen and note paper and thought a moment before she began writing: "MARGARET IN DYING CONDITION STOP ADVISE YOU COME AT ONCE STOP CHARLOTTE"

Charlotte read the message over. Then she preceded it with the name and address of her father at the Exchange Hotel in Winnipeg, her brother William at the pharmacy in Montreal, and her uncle Donald McDonald at the Senate in Ottawa. She got up and took the sheet of note paper into the kitchen. She gave it to George to take to the telegraph office.

Charlotte's father told her later that he received her telegram at a construction camp on the Whitemouth River, seventy-two miles northeast of Winnipeg. He had travelled day and night over almost 2,000 miles by horseback, handcar, stagecoach and railway to be by his wife's side when she died. He was five days late. Margaret lapsed into a coma early in the morning of Friday, February 16, the day after Charlotte had telegraphed her father. She died that afternoon.

Joseph went back out west a week after he buried his wife. Although there were letters, it was not until construction was shut down for Christmas that Charlotte learned first-hand about William and Caroline and how well her father's work was going. Her younger brother and his wife had arrived in Winnipeg at the end of May aboard the SS Minnesota. They had rented a modest but comfortable house a block or so from the business section on Main Street.

"William plans to open his drugstore next July," said David. "Right now he's helping to form a provincial association for pharmacists. He's just as enthusiastic as ever. More so, if that's possible."

Charlotte and her husband were preparing for bed. They

were enjoying their first private moments together since David had left for Manitoba in mid-January. Seated on the edge of the bed, David was watching his wife's nightly ritual of brushing out her hair.

"Tell me more about Lord and Lady Dufferin," said Charlotte.

Through the prime minister, Joseph had requested that the governor general and his wife preside over the ceremonial driving of the first spike on the Pembina Branch. While they were in Manitoba, he had brought the first locomotive into the North-West.

"They were pleased to have Joseph name it the Countess of Dufferin," said David.

"He and Charles arrived on a barge behind the SS Selkirk with the engine and tender, six flatcars and a caboose. William Luxton put out a special edition of his newspaper. The city's church bells and steam whistles set up a great racket. The best part, though, was when the Dufferins left on the SS Minnesota. You remember your father speaking of a man named James McKay?"

Charlotte nodded. She had finished brushing. She bowed her head, gathering her hair at the nape of her neck and reaching for a length of ribbon. "The man who took in the Indian woman and her child," she said.

"McKay was quite taken with the Dufferins. As a member of the Manitoba Cabinet, he said the official farewell. He went on with it even after the Minnesota cast off. He just missed getting dumped off the gangplank into the river."

Charlotte smiled. She could imagine the splash the big man would have made.

"McKay's famous dancing bear was on board. So was the bear's friend, a tame pig named Dick."

Charlotte laughed outright. "The Dufferins must think the West is a strange place," she said.

David had one piece of news that especially pleased her. Joseph had bought a fairly large house on Dagmar Street, not far from William and Caroline's own on McDermott. He was tired of the Exchange Hotel. It had been his home in Winnipeg for almost three years. The house was also a concession to his daughter. Charlotte had made it clear that she would not stay all year in Clinton while the men in her family, her husband in particular, spent the best part of it in Manitoba.

Charlotte passed the next two summers at her father's house in Winnipeg. The first year she travelled by rail to North Dakota and took the riverboat north, retracing the steps she had taken three years earlier with David and Margaret.

In that first summer, everything was going well. William was elected vice president of the Manitoba Pharmaceutical Association, which he had helped found. A few months later he opened his drugstore, the Medical Hall. It did well from the start, as Charlotte knew it would. People liked William. Charlotte had once joked to their stepmother that his engaging manner was as contagious as the German measles, if considerably more pleasant. In the spring, William and Caroline had a baby girl. They named her Ethel Maud Dora.

About the same time that he became a grandfather again, Joseph completed construction of the Pembina Branch. When Charlotte came west for the second summer, she was able to travel by rail from St. Paul, Minnesota, to St. Boniface. The trip took thirty-one hours. It had taken three days by riverboat.

Joseph had run into trouble with his work on the Canadian Pacific main line. Contract 15 involved laying track across the narrows at Cross Lake. It seemed bottomless. Rock ballast disappeared beneath the surface as fast as Joseph's crews could haul it. David said that the lake had never been surveyed properly. When his costs rose, Joseph had difficulty meeting payrolls. His men stopped work. There was strike violence. Joseph received little help from Ottawa. The government had changed the previous fall. The Conservatives were back in power. David had always been of the opinion that building railways was as much the business of politics as it was of construction. By mid-summer he felt that nothing short of a miracle could save Contract 15.

David and Charles decided that whatever happened they would stay in the West. David was buying up timber rights. His first lease was for 120 square miles of prime tamarack, jack pine and black spruce in the valley of the Whitemouth River. He advised Charlotte that he was scouting for others.

The last week in August, Charlotte took the train for St. Paul from St. Boniface Station. Her sister-in-law and the baby were travelling with her. Caroline was looking forward to showing off her daughter, whom her parents had never seen. She had another reason, which she confided to Charlotte. While she did not mind living in Winnipeg, Caroline missed the social and sophisticated city life she had known in Montreal.

Christmas Eve in Clinton, Charlotte regretted that the family was so scattered. David and Charles had decided to remain with Joseph in Manitoba to do what they could to help him salvage Contract 15. David was busy recruiting men to cut trees at a winter bush camp and to make up a river crew for the spring drive. Her brother William was living in a Winnipeg hotel while his wife and infant daughter visited with his in-laws in Montreal.

Charlotte shook her head at how things had changed since their stepmother had died. Life was never the same after the death of someone you loved. Margaret, God bless her and her commitment to all of them, had somehow always managed at meaningful times to keep her adoptive family together. Or perhaps, Charlotte reconsidered, it would have been different now. Maybe they had all been caught up in the process of growing apart as they grew older, and other obligations, other interests, intervened. The thought depressed her a little. At least she and Hanna and all the children were well and celebrating a family Christmas together in Clinton. This was reason enough, she told herself, to be thankful.

On her way up from the oyster barrel in the root cellar to the kitchen, she glanced at the clock on the parlour mantel board. Within the hour, depending on the degree of spitting and hissing the bird had yet to do, they would be sitting down to Christmas dinner. Charlotte had made sure there was plenty of everything for herself, Hanna, the ten children and the one man, her brother-in-law, who would be present. She hoped that Thomas and Mary Anne's two children would not be late.

Children? She smiled to herself. Mary Anne's daughter was seventeen, the same age as Bella. Her son was a year older than Kate. Josephine and William would have been insulted had they known that she thought of them as anything less than young adults! Especially Josie. Charlotte made a mental note to remember this. They mature so young, she mused; much sooner than we did. She smiled again over the tray of live oysters that she carried into the kitchen. She remembered her stepmother saying exactly the same thing when she and Mary Anne had been William and Josie's age. How we parents cling to the small hand of childhood, thought Charlotte. How we strain to keep it too long in our grasp. Always in vain.

While Bella and Hanna's daughter, Margaret, took turns basting the turkey, Kate helped the housegirl set the table. Charlotte's second eldest had turned fourteen just three months earlier. Kate the gossamer one, thought her mother. Uncertain as a butterfly and just as delicate. Always the first to catch an illness and the last to lose it. Just like Mary Anne.

When they heard the sleighbells at the front of the house, they thought it was Thomas and the two children. Charlotte followed Min into the entry hall. She stood by as her daughter opened the door.

"Mr. Straiton." Charlotte said.

The station agent was standing ill-at-ease. He had his railway cap in one hand and an envelope in the other. He held the envelope at his side, as though he hoped no one would notice it. Charlotte put this together with his cheerless expression and reflected that telegrams almost always meant bad news.

Alex Straiton cleared his throat and handed Charlotte the envelope. "I'm sorry to have to bring you this," he said. "Especially at Christmas."

Charlotte was touched by the man's concern. It was no secret that her father was having trouble out west. References to his problems at Cross Lake had been printed in *The New Era* and *The Toronto Globe*. "Thank you, Mr. Straiton," she said, managing a smile. "I appreciate your coming out on Christmas Eve, as I'm sure Mr. Whitehead would."

The station agent turned to go.

"A merry Christmas to you," Charlotte said.

Alex Straiton touched his fingers to his cap.

Charlotte closed the door and opened the envelope. The message inside was hand-written: "SADLY MUST ADVISE YOU THAT OUR GRANDDAUGHTER PASSED AWAY EARLY TODAY STOP HAVE TELEGRAPHED WILLIAM STOP FUNERAL SERVICE IS SATURDAY STOP PETER NICHOLSON"

"Mother?"

Charlotte did not hear her daughter. Caroline had written

her less than two weeks earlier that Ethel was ill, but not seriously. Was it the simple croup, as she had said? Or had it been something else? A more critical illness, perhaps. There was a kind of diphtheria called membranous croup. It was often fatal.

"Mother? What is it? What does it say?"

Min was standing at her elbow. Hanna had come out from the kitchen. They both read from her face that something was seriously wrong.

"It's a telegram from the Nicholsons," said Charlotte. "Your cousin Ethel has gone to be with God on Christmas Eve."

William stopped by in Clinton after the funeral. He was on his way back out west. Caroline had chosen to stay a while in Montreal. Charlotte's brother was still stunned by the death of his infant daughter. She had died at just seven months and eight days. It bothered Charlotte that William seemed to hold his wife at least partly responsible for their daughter's death.

"If only she hadn't insisted on going to Montreal."

"It could have happened anywhere," said Charlotte.

"Maybe not if she and the baby had stayed home."

Charlotte had to admit that this was possibly so. There had been an epidemic of simple croup in December among children in Montreal. The early symptoms were similar to membranous croup. It was possible that in some cases one might lead to the other. So little was known about the disease that until recently it had been thought that it was spread by swarming grasshoppers. Some still believed that it was.

Two pieces of news came out of Winnipeg in early spring.

Both were expected. In March, William was elected president of the Manitoba Pharmaceutical Association. A month later Ottawa cancelled Contract 15 with Charlotte's father. He was still camped at Cross Lake. Soon after, work was started up again under Michael Haney, a salaried superintendent of construction appointed by the government.

Near the end of May, Charlotte and Hanna surrounded themselves with shipping containers. Potbellied barrels obtained from John Pickett's cooperage stood about the house amid boxes of all sorts and sizes that they had begged from Clinton's shopkeepers. A special prize had been the half-dozen tea chests given to Charlotte by Shepherd and Cooper, grocers to the family for almost as many years as they had been in Clinton. Squat, square boxes with metal corners, sturdy enough to weather the China seas, they could not be accidentally rolled off platforms by railway freight handlers. Charlotte considered them even better than barrels for the safe packing of her precious breakables.

She took a dinner plate from the extravagant service her father had brought back from England. She paused nostalgically, turning it over in her hands. It was all so very long ago. Slowly, carefully, she wrapped the delicate china piece in a double sheet from a stack of newspapers. She placed it gently in the tea chest. She had always been fond of beautiful things. She picked up another plate.

Charlotte was alone in the house. The houseman and his wife had been given the afternoon off. Charles, Hanna and their children had gone to bid goodbye to their neighbours in Blyth – including old friends like John Clark at The Case is Altered Inn, where Charles had served as justice of the peace. David was off somewhere with their own children. Charlotte knew that he was trying to make up for his long absences in Manitoba. She had done the same when she came home from studying in Philadelphia.

Well, the family separations were almost ended now. They had decided that she and the children would live with Charles and his family in Joseph's house on Dagmar Street. David was planning to build a log house for them in Whitemouth after he built the sawmill. Until it was finished he would spend most of his weekends in Winnipeg. He hoped to have everything ready so that Charlotte and the children could move to Whitemouth not this summer but next.

Charles's plans were not as settled. Charlotte's elder brother was considering running for a seat on city council. He was also bidding on two contracts. One was to build a bridge across the Assiniboine River, not far from where it forked with the Red on the outskirts of Winnipeg. The other was to supply the city with firewood. He had also spoken of moving 100 miles or so west to be in on the start of a new prairie townsite. Charles had the uncomfortable feeling that Winnipeg was already getting too crowded.

Charlotte wrapped and packed the last of the dinner plates. She got up and walked to the dining-room window, which overlooked the flower garden. The shrub roses that her mother had brought from England were already in full bud. Charlotte cherished them. Her mother had said that they were direct descendants of the Yorkist emblem in the Wars of the Roses with the House of Lancaster. In the end the House of York had failed, but the rose had not. For more than 400 years it had flourished in old English gardens, its double blooms virgin white, their scent seductive. Charlotte's mother had taken cuttings from them before they sailed from England. Her daughter had made up her mind to do the same.

Charlotte was told that, while wild roses grew in the West, the Manitoba winter would be much too harsh for a civilized English rose. Even David, who knew how much it meant to her, told his wife that she would be wasting her time. Charlotte quietly kept her own counsel. Her Yorkist rose was an iron rose. She was convinced that it would not just survive the move to Whitemouth, but thrive in that primitive place. Just as she herself would.

CHAPTER ELEVEN

Winnipeg, Summer, 1880

CHARLOTTE AND HANNA and their families were well settled into the house on Dagmar Street by mid-July. Both mothers were pleased that all the children had soon found neighbourhood friends their own ages. This in turn had led Charlotte to set up the same kind of casual practice that she had known in Clinton.

Charlotte had learned from a neighbour that there were a number of women practising various types of medicine in Winnipeg. She had little doubt that the best at midwifery was Annie Power. As a young woman, the Widow Power had apprenticed at two well-respected lying-in hospitals: Norwich, in Norfolk, England, and Glasgow's St. Andrews. She had been delivering babies for twenty-five years. From what Charlotte could gather, the rest of the women were midwives of varying degrees of competence, herbalists, mystics and self-styled general practitioners who had never put in a day's formal study.

Many of Charlotte's new neighbours despaired of ever finding a qualified woman physician in Winnipeg. They soon discovered that Providence had finally provided one. Neighbourhood children, who heard it from Charlotte's and Hanna's children, told their mothers, who told their friends. Within a week of her arrival, Charlotte heard a knock at the door and opened it to a mother and her daughter. She guessed that the girl was about the same age as Min, who would be thirteen in October.

"Dr. Ross?"

Charlotte nodded acknowledgement. She looked enquiringly from the girl to her mother.

"This is my daughter, Patricia."

The girl, half-hidden behind her mother, shyly curtsied.

"She requires a doctor. May we come in?"

Charlotte had not intended to practise during the remaining ten months or so she would be spending in Winnipeg. She looked again at the girl standing on her doorstep. Her eyes were lacklustre, her skin pale. Charlotte opened the door wide. "Of course," she said. "Do please come in."

She examined the girl. While Patricia dressed, Charlotte talked with her mother. Her daughter had begun menstruating. Charlotte realized that in this family, as in most others, such things were not discussed, not even by a mother and her daughter. Patricia came into the parlour.

"I'll make tea," said Charlotte. Ending what had begun as a purely professional call with this unexpected gesture flattered the girl's mother. Charlotte brought her *Harper's Bazaar*, which had replaced *Godey's Lady's Book* as the arbiter of good taste and social behaviour. "I thought you might like to look through this while you're waiting," said Charlotte. She turned to the woman's daughter. "Would you care to help me, Patricia?"

164

Without waiting for an answer, Charlotte steered the girl from the parlour to the kitchen. She handed her the copper kettle from the back of the woodstove. "You hold this while I pump." Charlotte spoke to her quietly over the short strokes of the pump handle and the water that gushed from its spout. "What's happening isn't something that should make you afraid, or ashamed," she said. "And you're not sick." They talked while Charlotte made the tea and the girl set out the china and sugar cookies.

As Patricia and her mother were leaving, Charlotte prescribed for her. She told the girl to go to a neighbourhood butcher shop early every morning, when the killing was done, and ask for a cup of blood. She was to drink this. Charlotte wanted to see her again in a week's time.

The blood was for the treatment of pernicious anemia, a condition sometimes brought on by the menstrual start. The talk with Patricia was to help her understand that menstruation was simply one of the rites of passage to becoming a woman.

On the last Thursday in July, the sheriff of Winnipeg died accidentally. It happened just after midnight. Richard Power was returning an escaped prisoner from Rat Portage. The two men stepped from the dock at St. Boniface into a small boat to cross the river to Winnipeg. One of them lost his footing. Sheriff Power and highwayman Mike Carroll both drowned.

Charlotte later reflected on how this tragedy touched her life. The sheriff's mother was Annie Power, the woman who had been trained in midwifery in England and Scotland and practised in Winnipeg. His wife was Augusta, the grown-up little Indian girl that James and Margaret McKay had taken into their home fifteen years earlier. Charlotte remembered her father speaking of the McKays' kindness to the girl and her mother during her visit west with David and Margaret. Charlotte never would have believed then that she and the woman the McKays named Harriett would one day meet and become good friends. Their relationship began on the Sunday morning of the state funeral for Sheriff Power.

Harriett and her daughter had grown apart over the years. As much as she had been accepted into the household, Harriett had always served as a nanny to the McKays' three children and her own daughter. She had never been a member of the family, as Augusta was. Augusta was legally entitled to call herself a McKay. Her mother had simply assumed the surname because she needed one. James McKay had had a lot to do with arranging Augusta's marriage to the promising young law-enforcement officer. Richard Power was also a horse officer with the Winnipeg Infantry Company at Fort Osborne Barracks. After Augusta's marriage, she and her mother had grown even further apart.

Both the McKays had died the previous year, Margaret quickly and unexpectedly near the end of February, James at the beginning of December after a lingering illness. Charlotte's father had been McKay's friend and business associate. Joseph had brought four more locomotives into Manitoba after his first, the Countess of Dufferin. Most were construction-work engines. *Bullgines* he called them. He had named them all. One had been named the James McKay.

When McKay died, Harriett had stayed on at Deer Lodge to look after the two boys, James and Angus. Their sister, Jane Dallas, had become a boarder at St. Mary's Academy, a Winnipeg teaching convent run by the Sisters of the Holy Names of Jesus and Mary.

Just before noon, Charlotte's father and Harriett arrived at the house on Dagmar Street in a covered coach and pair. The carriage was driven by a liveryman, smartly suited in grey with a matching cape and a black silk top hat. They were on their way back from the requiem high mass and funeral for Sheriff Power at St. Mary's Cathedral. In a chivalrous act that Charlotte found typical of her father, Joseph had hired the carriage for Harriett, and had offered to be her escort. He had told Charlotte the previous evening that he intended to stop by on the drive back to Deer Lodge.

The woman that her father ushered into the parlour appeared to Charlotte to be not much older than her own thirty-seven years. She was fashionably, if severely, dressed. A small hat with a veil was perched on midnight-black hair parted in the middle and tied back in a tight bun. Behind the veil, she had dark eyes and high cheekbones, skin that was smooth and not quite russet. Her mouth, slightly downturned at the corners, lifted when she smiled, as she did now.

Charlotte's father introduced them.

"It's a great pleasure to meet you, Mrs. Ross."

"And you, Miss McKay."

"Harriett, please."

Charlotte liked the gentle smile, warm and assured. "Then you must call me Charlotte," she said.

"I thought you might put on a pot of tea," said Joseph. "This has all been very difficult for Harriett." His voice, like his manner, was solicitous.

"I'll put the kettle on," said Charlotte. She excused herself and went to the kitchen.

Hanna had not yet returned from walking the children to where they could watch the funeral procession through the city, past flags flown at half-mast. Led by Father Albert Lacombe, Sheriff Power's coffin was borne on a gun carriage. Behind came his riderless horse, his boots up-ended in the stirrups, followed by the Winnipeg Infantry Company battery band. Annie Power, Augusta and her two small children, Mary Adelaide and Michael Buhan, occupied the first carriage in the cortège.

While she waited for the kettle to boil, Charlotte rejoined her father and their guest in the parlour. She walked directly to Harriett and sat down beside her. "Augusta has my prayers and my sympathy," she said. She took one of Harriett's hands in her own. "As do you. God bless you both, and the dear children, too."

Only Harriett's eyes changed expression. They warmed to Charlotte's words and the hands that covered hers. Whatever she felt about the death of her daughter's husband, she remained stoic. Harriett was a Santee. Seventeen years earlier, in the Minnesota Uprising, the Santee, under Chief Whitecap, had been crushed by the United States Cavalry. Most of the survivors had fled north to Manitoba and the North-West Territory, which lay west of it. Harriett and her five-year-old daughter had been among them.

A little more than a month remained until Jane Dallas was to re-enter St. Mary's Academy, and Harriett was to take the girl's two brothers to live with relatives in Montreal. During that time Harriett was a frequent visitor at the house on Dagmar, sometimes arriving with Joseph, often as a guest of her daughter. A week before she left Winnipeg with James and Angus, Charlotte picked her up at Deer Lodge to take afternoon tea with Caroline.

When his wife returned from Montreal in late spring, William had found a house on Smith Street, not far from St. Mary's Cathedral. The area was pleasantly residential, quite removed from the commercial end of town. He and Caroline had agreed that a change of neighbourhood, a street swept clean of memories, might be good for both of them. Although almost eight months had passed, Caroline had not yet come to terms with the death of her daughter. Depending on her mood, she vacillated between blaming her husband for moving them to Winnipeg and herself for returning with Ethel Maud to Montreal. Although Harriett and Augusta were only estranged, Charlotte realized, as she grew to know Harriett better, that the loss was no less wrenching for her. She thought that meeting this woman who had learned acceptance might be a good prescription for her sister-in-law. As different as the circumstances were, both women had lost a daughter.

Charlotte had arranged the tea under the pretext of introducing Harriett, who had never been to Montreal, to someone who knew it well. She was pleased to see that Caroline was in good spirits. As her sister-in-law poured, Charlotte explained the reason for their visit. "My friend wants to know everything you think she should know," she said, "before she leaves next week."

Caroline laughed. She handed each of her guests a cup of tea before replying. "I am not sure," she said, "that we have the time!"

Charlotte was worried about William. The death of his infant daughter had been as much of a blow to him as it had been to Caroline. She suspected that he had not looked after himself as well as he might have during his wife's lengthy stay with her parents in Montreal.

Charlotte and Hanna were busy the first Saturday in September. They were getting their children ready for the opening of Central School, where the subjects taught were reading, writing and "figuring." Caroline came for Charlotte in mid-morning. William had developed a cough a few days earlier. It had worsened, and now he had a fever. A sharp pain whenever he coughed made him clutch at his chest with both hands. Caroline told Charlotte that she was afraid her husband was coming down with pneumonia.

Since the day of the tea with Harriett, Charlotte had not seen much of her sister-in-law. She reflected on this, not speaking.

While Caroline drove, she kept her eyes on her horse's flanks and the narrow streets. Charlotte addressed her profile. "How have you both been? Has William been generally well? Until now, I mean?"

"He's been working very hard." Caroline gave Charlotte a sidelong glance. "I think perhaps overdoing it. He's so ambitious to open another drugstore, and another one after that." She was silent a moment. "Then there's the Pharmaceutical Association. He takes his responsibilities as president very seriously."

While she spoke, their horse had slowed to a walk. Caroline flicked the reins and clucked impatiently, urging the animal into a reluctant trot.

"There seems to be no end to the late evenings," she said. She glanced again at her sister-in-law. She was suddenly defensive. "Not that I mind, of course."

Charlotte nodded. She knew that of course Caroline minded. She was aware that her brother put in long hours, hoping to expand his Medical Hall into a successful chain. At the same time, she wondered if the frequent meetings, which Caroline told her usually took place in the Grand Central Hotel, were as pharmaceutical as they were social. This was where William had lived while his wife was in Montreal. She had ruefully admitted on her return that he would not have been William had he not been immensely popular and made a great many new friends.

William was propped up in bed. She saw with some satisfaction that he was not now feeling like the life of the party. She chided herself for this uncharitable thought. She hoped the smile that it brought on would be interpreted simply as bedside manner. It was.

"No one should come so cheerfully into a sickroom," said William. "Especially not a doctor, knowing that the patient is already knocking at death's door."

Charlotte was not deceived by her brother's bravado. She knew he was dreading his next fit of coughing. She set her medical bag on the bureau and took out her stethoscope. "Undo your nightshirt."

"You forget I'm a pharmacist," William grumbled. "I don't need a doctor to tell me I'm sick, or what to do about it."

Charlotte sat by his side. She felt his forehead for fever. "Physicians write the prescriptions. Pharmacists fill them." She withdrew her hand. "More to the point, younger brothers do what their older sisters tell them."

Before she could unbutton his nightshirt, William began coughing. He leaned over the bedside, spitting rusted sputum into a washbowl. The pain caused him to cry out. Charlotte put her arms around him. She made soothing sounds and stroked his head until the spasm subsided. William lay back against the pillows, exhausted. Charlotte shook down her thermometer and slipped it under his tongue. This time he did not protest when she opened his nightshirt and moved the bell of her stethoscope across his chest. She listened for the sound of leather rubbing against leather that would confirm her initial diagnosis.

"Can you take a deep breath?"

William nodded. He stopped short at the stitch in his side.

"That's good."

Charlotte removed the thermometer. It read two degrees over the oral norm of 98.6. Caroline was watching anxiously from the foot of the bed. Charlotte got up and walked to her medical bag. She exchanged her stethoscope for a hypodermic syringe and a vial of cloudy liquid. "Your husband has pleurisy," she said.

She removed the stopper from the vial and drew a measure of liquid into the syringe. "The membranes that line the lungs and chest are inflamed. Breathing, or worse still coughing, rubs one against the other. It can be very painful." She put the vial back in her bag and returned to William's bedside, holding the hypodermic needle upright. "The membranes are called pleura."

Charlotte bared her brother's arm. She deftly inserted the needle and emptied the syringe. She ignored his exaggerated "ouch."

"I've given him an injection of heroin," she said to Caroline. "That should kill the pain and keep the coughing down. He'll need complete rest in bed. For now he's on a liquid diet; nothing but water, juices, gruels and broths." She walked to the bureau and returned the syringe to her medical bag.

"I can't just close up shop," said William.

Charlotte snapped the bag shut. "Be sensible. Your present condition is more painful than it is serious. That doesn't mean it won't get worse if you don't take care of yourself."

"I'll see that he does," Caroline promised.

"Good. Take his temperature every three hours or so. If it rises significantly, send for me. If not, I'll look in again this time tomorrow."

Charlotte picked up her bag and prepared to leave with Caroline. "We'll stop by and tell Mr. Luxton you're indisposed for the next few days. I'm sure he'll put something in his newspaper."

"The next few days?" William echoed.

"At least," Charlotte said firmly.

Her first fall in Manitoba, Charlotte fell in love with its subtle farewell to summer. Where she had lived in Ontario and Quebec the trees held Mardi Gras before the Lenten winter, costumed in festive reds and golds. The Manitoba fall came softly as a moccasin, branch-brushing the land with rusts and mauves and muted yellows. Sometimes, when everyone was somewhere else, Charlotte took her five-year-old son for a buggy ride along the river road. She would bundle up herself and Hales in a buffalo robe, the air as fresh as the sky was blue. They would stop by the empty river and watch geese fly overhead in point formation, filling the horizon south with their *basso profundo* farewells.

Sometimes, standing on her front porch in late evening, Charlotte could hear the geese but not see them. Their dark passage made silhouettes against the harvest moon that her mother used to say was God's lantern. Charlotte's thoughts would fly to Whitemouth and the house of logs that David would be starting in the spring. After a while she would shiver a little, feeling the impatient chill of winter. She would walk back inside, past the graceful mahogany table in the entry hall with its small sterling tray for calling cards.

Christmas came on with a confused rush. As Hanna put it, so much was happening that nothing seemed to get done. Charles was building a bridge across the Assiniboine River, and supplying the city with firewood. Charlotte's father was heavily involved in the real-estate boom that had begun nine years earlier with the start on the railway west. William was fully recovered from the attack of pleurisy he had suffered. He had expanded his shelves at the Medical Hall to include imported perfumes and other small gifts, and was having his best season yet.

David made it home for the holidays on Christmas Eve. He and a Cree Indian guide had been timber cruising to the northwest, along the shores of Lake Winnipegosis. Charlotte's husband was interested in a prime stand of trees covering some fifty-five square miles on Birch Island. On the day they reached it, his guide decoded wilderness signs that told him they could expect a sharp drop in the already numbing temperature. The previous Christmas Eve had been the coldest anyone could remember. The temperature had plunged to fifty-five below. David and his guide started for home that same afternoon.

This was Charlotte's first prairie winter. She decided that the whetstone Arctic winds that gave the cold its cutting edge and the heavy snows that threatened to bury them were a mixed blessing. Because work was frozen to a standstill, David was home for Christmas. So was Charles. Charlotte's father was not.

Contract 15 was near completion. Under the terms of his financial settlement with Ottawa, it was important that he return east. From something he said, Charlotte was aware that her father also planned a side trip on the Quebec, Montreal, Ottawa and Occidental Railway, a luxury express linking the capital with Quebec and its sea lanes to Europe. It was a reference to James McKay's two boys and his interest in seeing how they were getting along in Montreal.

The telephone lines that were strung up in Winnipeg in May convinced Charlotte's older brother that Winnipeg was becoming too "establishment" for him. The switch was thrown on the twenty-second. The next day Charles shipped out with a partner, Frank Myer, to start a real-estate and building-supply company at a settlement called Brandon, about 100 miles west. Hanna had agreed to remain in Winnipeg with their daughter and two sons until Charles had picked a site and built a house for them.

Charlotte went with her sister-in-law and the children to see him off aboard the SS North-West. It was loaded to the gunwales with lumber. The paddlewheeler backed off from the dock. In midstream it churned into forward and started up the Red towards the Assiniboine. Once out of sight, it would follow the river's meander west to the new townsite. Charlotte looked downriver towards the Louise Bridge. Men were still working on its three sections of superstructure. They were strung out like an open bracelet between the Winnipeg and St. Boniface banks of the Red River. Scheduled to be completed in less than three weeks, it would carry the first train to cross the river into Winnipeg. Pulling it would be the Countess of Dufferin.

As soon as possible after this, Charlotte planned to pack her family, her furniture and all the boxes and barrels of belongings they had brought west with them onto the train for Whitemouth. She was not concerned that David had been so busy at the mill that the house he had promised was still unfinished. Nor did she care that because of this he was not expecting them until some time in mid-summer. She intended to have their sixth child, the one she had been carrying since Christmas, at home in Whitemouth.

Charlotte and her family arrived at Manitoba Railway Station No. 1 early in the morning on the last Wednesday in June. Because she had ordered that a special railway car be fitted out for them, this was the soonest they could leave for Whitemouth after the first bridge crossing two weeks earlier.

Their livery carriage drew up to the station platform near a group of railway sectionmen. The men were looking at one of two flatcars coupled between the last passenger coach and the caboose. Behind the usual load of boxes and barrels, six passenger seats were bolted to its deck in pairs.

Bella felt the sectionman watching as the liveryman alighted and extended a steadying arm. She placed a hand on his arm and stepped down. "This," she murmured, "is going to be positively embarrassing."

Charlotte glanced at her sharply. "Nonsense," she said. "The railway people thought it was a wonderful idea."

Bella was not convinced. She looked down as she crossed the platform to the train. As she lifted her skirts ankle-high to step onto the flatcar, one of the men said something. Someone sniggered.

Charlotte turned on them. "Have you men nothing better to do than act the fool?" Her voice was as hard as a section foreman's.

The men looked sheepish. They moved off down the platform. Charlotte turned her back on them.

"The train should be leaving soon," she said. "We'd best take our seats."

Charlotte had arranged both to ride and to ship their belongings aboard the two flatcars. At the front of the first stood a stylish new phaeton. Its harness shafts were thrust forward like bowsprits, as though it was ready to proceed to Whitemouth under full sail.

In a busy final week of shopping, Charlotte had bought the convertible four-wheeler at Christopher Montgomery's Northwest Works. Securely lashed down behind the two-horse carriage was the handsomely worked piano Joseph had presented to Margaret as a homecoming gift. He had given it to Charlotte as a memento of her stepmother. The rest of the furniture had come from their house on the banks of the Bandon River, where they had lived when they were first married, and from their house in Montreal. Carefully stacked and secured, it included a five-tiered mahogany and glass whatnot that Charlotte had safeguarded by having it crated in Clinton. Whether she was moving from one room to another, or from east to west, Charlotte made sure that none of her precious things got broken.

The front end of the second flatcar was loaded with the boxes and barrels of silver, china, embroidered linens and other household goods that she had packed with such care in Clinton. Behind these were the passenger seats that she had ordered bolted to the deck. Charlotte did not want her family to travel to Whitemouth by coach. From her visit to her father's construction camp five summers earlier, she knew what sort of men would be riding the train to Cross Lake. She did not expect either their language or their conduct to make any of them suitable travelling companions for her young son and four daughters. She was also loathe to place them in close quarters with journeymen railway workers. Moving from place to place, and often less than fastidious, they were too often carriers of contagious diseases.

Charlotte had outfitted her family well for their trip by flatcar to join their father. She had spent a great deal of time with Miss Beswetherick at Alexander and Bryce, the ladies' import shop just a few doors down from William's drugstore. She and her three older daughters wore variations of a low-crowned silk hat secured by a knotted chiffon scarf. A full veil was added to keep the cinders from their eyes. Over full-length bouffant dresses they wore English dolmans – serge mantles with flaps for sleeves. Carrie wore a wool dress to the tops of her high-button black leather boots, Hales a two-piece serge suit. They both were hatted in broad-brimmed straws, banded with ribbon.

"Hold onto your hats!" shouted Charlotte.

She knew now why her father called them bullgines. On an open flatcar the engine's bellow was louder, its charge more headlong, its snort sootier than Charlotte had ever imagined from her Pullman palace car. The loose couplings between the cars gave and pulled like fractured elbows. The cars jerked from side to side, finally straightening out on the approach to the Louise Bridge. It launched them over the river. Just as Charlotte thought they might drop in a shower of cinders into the Red, it landed them safely on the other side. The waters that swirled beneath had seemed giddily close, still swollen and muddy from the late spring run-off.

Charlotte enjoyed the rest of the trip. Broad stretches of forest, broken here and there by land cleared for farms and small settlements, gave her a sense of the new life that she was about to begin. She was not happy to be retiring from practice. She had put too much into her profession to lay it to rest, even with the promise of eventual resurrection, without a small sense of dying herself. In this she was aware that she had little choice. In Whitemouth she knew that she would not be a doctor, but a woman living in a world of men.

Their train's shrill approach warnings were lost in the shriek of the noon steam whistle at David's sawmill. It stood just east of town on the banks of the Whitemouth River. As the railway station came into view, Charlotte saw that it was just a boxcar without wheels. On a spur track, a crew from the mill stopped off-loading lumber onto a flatcar from a horse-drawn wagon. David was among them. The train slowed, boiler heaving, drive-wheels rasping in a cloud of steam. One of the men pointed their way and said something to Charlotte's husband. David turned and looked.

"There's your father," said Charlotte.

Hales and his sisters hadn't seen him yet. They were returning the curious stares of a scattering of men, most of them part of a railway section gang, who had begun unpacking their lunches by the boxcar station.

"Where?" asked Hales.

Charlotte got up and bent over her son. She put her arms around him, facing him in the right direction. "Over there," she said. "Loading lumber."

Min waved and called out to her father. Her sisters joined in.

David dropped one hand to the floor of the mill wagon and vaulted to the ground. He took his time, walking deliberately towards them. The workmen sat eating their sandwiches. They watched in silence. David stopped in front of Charlotte and looked up at her. "You're a few weeks early," he said.

"Yes."

"I should have known you might be."

"Yes.

David reached up and lifted her down from the flatcar. "There's still work to be done on the house," he said.

"We can help."

Hales and Carrie clambered down the short ladder at one end of the flatcar and ran to their father. Min descended cautiously, holding her cumbersome skirts clear while Bella and Kate waited their turn. David caught his wife's glance at the silently watch-ing workmen. Amusement tugged at the corners of his mouth. "It's not just your coming by flatcar," he said. "You're the first white women they've seen in Whitemouth."

CHAPTER TWELVE

Whitemouth, Summer, 1881

*C*HARLOTTE WAS AWAKENED by a finger of sunshine that found a chink between the logs of her unfinished house and poked her in the eye. She blinked. Then she came slowly and smiling to her new surroundings. The solid look and good smell of the freshly cut and peeled timbers appealed to her. She knew she would appreciate them even more come next winter. Chinked with mud and straw, heated by the big cast-iron stove in the kitchen, they would provide the warmth of a thick wool blanket against wind and cold.

Charlotte raised herself on one elbow and looked at her husband. He was still sleeping. He and a handful of his men had worked late into the night hauling their things to the house after unloading them from the flatcars. They had begun by hitching a two-horse team to the phaeton. David had driven Charlotte and the two younger children over the bumpy road that led the half mile along the Whitemouth River to their new home. Called a corduroy road, it was made of logs laid side by side and covered with moss. Min and her two older sisters had followed with the first wagon-load of barrels and boxes. When Charlotte had not been seeing to the unloading and placing of each new load of furniture, she and the children were busy unpacking. By near midnight they were finally moved in, to everyone's satisfaction but Charlotte's. She was still trying things here and there, critically standing back to study the effect, until David suggested that she begin re-arranging again in the morning.

Charlotte got out of bed, being careful not to awaken her husband. She put on a night robe and went into the kitchen. She lit the fire that Bella had laid just before retiring so they could have their early morning tea. She decided not to awaken their eldest daughter until it was time for her to help with breakfast. Although their new home was unlike any they had ever lived in, Charlotte was pleased. David had done well. He had built the house on high ground at the edge of the forest. It overlooked a duck-shaped bend in the Whitemouth River with the mill at its tailfeathers. It was much larger than she had expected. Its thick walls were peeled on the inside and rose to a steeply pitched, vertical-slab roof. Its floors were smoothly planked of mouse-proof tamarack. The doors and windows were well-fitted and neatly trimmed. It had a big kitchen with a good view of the mill and the river below. The parlour and the dining room were combined into one very large room. There were five bedrooms, one of which was to serve as a guest room. Behind the house, land had been cleared for both a flower and a vegetable garden. There was a stable with a hay mow, a chicken coop, stalls for four horses, and storage for the phaeton, a wagon and a sleigh.

"What have you planned for this morning?"

David had drunk two cups of tea from the large pot Charlotte had brewed earlier and set on the back of the cookstove. Then he and Hales, as the two men in the family, sat down to a breakfast that Bella and Kate prepared and served – oatmeal porridge, eggs and bacon, wild raspberry jam, home-baked bread and freshly churned butter. Charlotte had joined them for a cup of tea, buttering and spreading jam thinly on one of the thick slices of bread that Min toasted over the open fire. She had baked the bread herself and brought it from Winnipeg.

"I have a few thoughts on the furniture," she said. "I can do some arranging while the girls iron and hang the curtains. Then I really must get my rose canes into the ground."

David got up from the table. "I still doubt they'll make it through the winter."

"We'll see."

David shrugged. "When you're through planting, you might like to take a walk down and see the mill."

"I'm looking forward to it."

Bella put off buttering a slice of toast, the knife poised. "May I come, too?"

"Certainly," said her father. "All of you, if you like."

David was flattered by his older daughter's interest in his work. He was proud of the mill he had built and how well it was doing.

"Only when you've finished your chores," said her mother. "New as it is, I want this house scrubbed from top to bottom."

"Mo-ther!" The recurring spectre of a paring knife and two wash buckets brought a pout to Bella's lips. Meant as a silent appeal to her father, it was wasted on him.

"None of that," said David. "You'll do as your mother says. All five of you."

His voice was stern, but as he walked to the kitchen door he favoured his eldest daughter with a covert wink. She reminded him in so many ways of the young woman he had married twenty years earlier. As well as her good looks, he had always admired Bella for having the same kind of spunk that her mother had. She had already asked him if she could work at the mill. This was out of the question, of course. Still, he hadn't given her an outright no. Perhaps there was something not actually in the mill itself, he had hinted, but yet to do with the mill.

"Anything!" Bella had said.

David had been charmed as always by so surprising a show of manliness in this daughter, who was so much a woman. He had promised to give it some thought.

The stationary steam engine that was the heart of the mill was started up at exactly the same time each morning, six days a week. Its beat began with a couple of lively blasts on its steam whistle. This was not long after the early man at the mill had filled the boiler with river water, built a crib of kindling and split logs in the firebox, and put a match to it. The shrill whistle told everyone within a good three miles upriver and down that it was precisely eight o'clock by David Ross's gold pocket watch. The workday at the mill had begun.

From where she knelt in the flower garden, Charlotte could hear the steady, percussive chug of the steam engine. It was punctuated by the regular shriek of steel ripping into wood. Because of the noise, she was thankful that David had built their home on ground as high and as far away from the mill as he had. She dug a deep hole for the first of her York rose canes and soaked it down well. She set the cane so its sleeping roots would come awake unbent, with room to stretch. The she gently filled and packed earth around it. The newly cleared and dug soil slipped through her fingers like the silk of her petticoat, wonderfully enriched by centuries of fallen leaves and tamarack needles. Charlotte had been told as a child that the tamarack was the only evergreen that shed its coat each fall. While clearing land at The Corners, her father had said that it was not only mouse-proof, but it was also best for fence posts and railway ties. It was splintery tough and had its own oils for preservative. Her father had called it the eastern larch.

Charlotte gave the mound around her first planting a final pat for good luck. She had many memories of early good times at The Corners, when her Yorkshire mother was still living and her father was too young ever to grow old. She tipped her pail of water, wetting down the mound so the roots of the rose would become one with the soils. She told herself that if the child she was expecting in September were a son, she would name him Joseph Whitehead Ross. She thought about this for a moment. Then she nodded her satisfaction with her decision and set down the pail. She was careful not to spill a drop.

Water, Charlotte had learned just that morning, was to be a problem in their new home. Well, she corrected herself, not exactly a problem, not when a whole river of it was stretched out beneath her kitchen window. More like a great deal of hard work. David told her at breakfast that they got their water by filling barrels at the riverbank. These were then lashed to a stone boat, a platform of boards on heavy wood runners, which was hauled by a two-horse team up the steep, winding road to the house.

Charlotte could hear her three older daughters filling pails from a barrel, and emptying them into the large cauldron on top of the woodstove. She had cautioned Kate not to overdo it, and Bella to see that she didn't. Carrie and Hales were in and out of the house, fetching wood to build a fire big enough to bring the cauldron to boiling. Scrubbing down the whole house, while the two younger children kept them in clean wash-cloths and mop-cloths, would occupy Bella and her sisters for the better part of the day. Charlotte began vigorously digging another hole. She did not just evangelize the belief, impressed on her by her mother, that idle hands make work for the devil. She actively practised it.

From his first day on Contract 15, David had looked after members of his father-in-law's crews who fell ill or were injured. Joseph had chosen him for the job because he knew of his son-in-law's interest in medicine. When father and husband had argued over the wisdom of Charlotte's decision to go to Philadelphia, David had pointed out that had his own steps taken a different path he might have studied to become a doctor himself. For the next three years, David had been all the doctor there was between end of track and St. Boniface Hospital. He had often given first aid to sick or hurt workers before they were bundled onto a handcar or, if their condition was not critical, put aboard one of "Whitehead's trains." As a layman, David had done well. This did not diminish his relief that a real doctor had finally come to Whitemouth.

Charlotte finished soaking down the last of her rose canes. She up-ended the pail to get all the water. Min appeared at the kitchen door.

"There's a man here from the mill," she called out.

Charlotte nodded, straightening, brushing the soil from her skirts.

"He says father wants you to come with your medical bag."

Charlotte set the empty pail on the back stoop and entered the house. Bella was standing by the open front door. She was holding a paring knife in one hand and her mother's black leather bag in the other.

The man at the door nodded. "Lewis McCall, ma'am. Mr. Ross asks that you come down to the mill."

Charlotte took the bag from Bella. "Has there been an accident?"

"No, ma'am. One of the men's down with something. He's real sick."

McCall was standing with his cap in his hands, working a hoop with his fingers. "It's maybe the fever," he said.

That told Charlotte why he was visibly uneasy. "The fever" was typhoid. It was common where carriers came and went among casual workers and drinking water was often contaminated. Sometimes called autumnal fever, it was most prevalent in the fall. Water supplies were usually lower than in spring and summer, and not as fresh. The mortality rate was high.

David's office was just inside the entrance to the mill. It was large enough for a desk and chair, a squat, iron safe and one other chair. A bench along one wall provided seating for three more visitors, four in a squeeze. When Charlotte entered, it was occupied by two mill workers she guessed to be in their mid-twenties. One of them half-lay along the bench, slouched in the arms of the other. A third and slightly older man that Charlotte saw was David's foreman was seated across the desk from her husband.

"Here's the doctor now," said David.

The sick man turned and lifted his head to look. It took him a moment to focus on Charlotte through eyes hazed with fever. He choked out a protest and tried to get to his feet. His friend tightened his hold to keep him from falling off the bench.

"Be still, Peter!" he said. "You're too sick to be getting up."

Peter made another attempt to free himself. It was even feebler this time. He fell back, exhausted. "She's a woman," he said hoarsely.

Charlotte put her medical bag on her husband's desk. She pretended she hadn't heard as she snapped open its catches and took out her thermometer. The mill foreman set his empty chair by the bench.

"She's a woman!" the sick man said again, louder this time, as though his friend might be deaf as well as blind.

Charlotte was standing over them, prepared to sit and start her examination.

The sick man's friend looked embarrassed for him. "For God's sake, you may be dying from the fever," he said. "You better take whatever help you can get. Wherever it's from."

Charlotte sat and smiled reassuringly. "It's Peter, is it?"

"Peter Hall," David said from behind his desk.

Charlotte reached out her thermometer. "Well, Mr. Hall, if we can raise our head just a little."

His friend raised it for him.

"Good." Charlotte shook down the thermometer and slipped it under his tongue. When she took hold of his wrist he tried to pull away. Her fingers on his pulse and her thumb on the back of his wrist made an unyielding vice. She checked his pulse against the sweep-second hand of the gold watch she wore pinned to her blouse. His beat was slightly higher than normal. Charlotte attributed this partly to his agitation with her. She addressed his friend.

"How long has Mr. Hall been feeling unwell?"

"About a week. It's been that long since he first mentioned it."

Charlotte pressed her hand against the sick man's abdomen. "Does that hurt?"

Peter Hall fixed his eyes on the ceiling. "No, ma'am." He muttered around the thermometer in his mouth, shivering a little. His nose was runny. He brushed at it with a clenched fist.

"Have you been having nose bleeds?"

"No, ma'am."

"Loss of appetite?"

He shook his head.

"Nausea?"

He frowned. "Ma'am?"

"Have you felt like you wanted to throw up?"

"No, ma'am."

Charlotte took the thermometer from his mouth. It showed two degrees above normal. "Have you been bothered by headaches?"

He nodded.

"Pains in your legs and back?"

He nodded again.

"Constipation or diarrhea?"

"Ma'am?"

"Has your bowel been stopped up, or have you been having frequent and loose movements?"

Peter Hall gagged. The eyes that had been fixed on the ceiling squeezed shut. His mortified "no, ma'am" was whispered.

Charlotte spoke briskly to his friend. "Unbutton his shirt."

Peter Hall groaned.

Charlotte bared his chest, examined it, then closed his shirt again. She pressed the fingers of both hands against the lymphatic glands in his neck, just below the jaw. "Have you a sore throat?"

He nodded.

Satisfied, Charlotte got up and put the thermometer back in her bag. With her back to the two men on the bench she smiled at her husband.

"Well?" said David.

Charlotte turned and looked down at Peter Hall. She knew that both he and his friend were expecting the worst. "It would appear," she said, "that you have nothing more serious than German measles."

While she spoke lightly, Charlotte did not underestimate the discomfort caused by rubella, as it was medically named, or its potential dangers. She was relieved that Peter Hall did not have typhoid fever. At the same time, her examination told her that he had "sickened for the disease." This was said to be the case when the symptoms were present but the disease itself had not developed. Bottled up inside, it made the patient more miserable and subject to complications, such as pneumonia, than if the disease had run its usual course.

Charlotte ordered her patient put on a makeshift pallet in one of the mill wagons and driven to Whitemouth. He and his friend shared a room at Mrs. Enright's boarding house. She asked that he get Peter Hall back home and into bed. She told him to move to another room until the danger of infection was past.

Charlotte walked up the hill to the house. She got a handful of pumpkin seeds from among the roots, seeds and leaf herbs that were bagged in butter muslin and hung to dry in the kitchen pantry. She was aware that there were some things Indians knew and which weren't taught in medical school. Her mother had learned of simple herbal aids and remedies, like the benefits of salicin crystals from willow bark as a pain reliever, when they had lived at The Corners. Neighbouring Ojibwa had taught her, too, about pumpkin seeds. Charlotte put the handful of seeds into a pot of water on the cookstove. While Bella harnessed the horses to the phaeton, Charlotte simmered a broth that would bring out the pinkish-red rubella spots on her patient's face and chest.

Charlotte had not expected to practise again until the railway west was completed and there were homestead women and children who needed medical care. On the drive to Mrs. Enright's boarding house, she thought it a strange trick of fate that her first patient in Whitemouth was neither.

Charlotte was mildly amused by the men lounging in the hallway. Seated at Peter Hall's bedside, spooning him the broth she had brewed, she could feel their eyes on her back. She had noticed them when Mrs. Enright brought the wash cloth and basin of warm water she requested. The landlady had left after setting the tin wash basin down on a table by the bed. Never before had she allowed her own house rule to be broken that no woman, other than herself, was permitted in her bachelor-workingmen's rooms. She had been prepared to hover. She had retreated downstairs only after Charlotte thanked her on a pleasant but unmistakeable note of dismissal. Mrs. Enright's backward glance had clearly said that she did not approve. Her final statement had been to leave the bedroom door open behind her.

Charlotte spooned the last of the broth from the bowl and set it down by the wash basin. She tested the water for tepidness, soaked the wash cloth, and wrung it out. She gently bathed Peter Hall's face. She put the cloth back in the basin and unbuttoned his shirt. He did not draw back in protest as he had at the mill. The jolting wagon ride home that had kept him from slipping into a coma had given him time to think through his fever. Dismay at being treated by a woman doctor had given way to relief that she was there to help him. As she stripped off his shirt, Charlotte remembered her audience. She got up and crossed the floor. She shut the door gently but firmly on the gallery in the hallway.

Mrs. Enright soon discovered that Charlotte's visits to her boarder's upstairs bedroom would continue until he was well again.

She returned early the next morning with a covered pot of gruel. She instructed that the basins of warm water she used to sponge down her patient be prepared twice daily. The rubella spots came out on Peter Hall's face and the rest of his body three days later. His fever broke. After four more days the spots faded and flaked away. Peter Hall recovered nicely.

The knock at the front door of the Ross house was a tentative one. It was the sort of knock made by someone who wants to make his presence known without disturbing anyone. Bella heard it because she was already in the entry hall, ready to leave for her job at the mill. She answered the knock and returned to the kitchen. Charlotte was lingering over a cup of tea while Kate and Min cleared the breakfast dishes.

"There's someone to see you, Mother," said Bella. "I think it's one of the men from the mill." She frowned at the kitchen clock. "I have to run."

Charlotte glanced at the clock. It was a good ten minutes yet before her husband would consult his pocket watch and bring a shriek to the virgin silence.

"You've no need to rush," she said to Bella. She rose to go to the door, taking her cup and saucer with her. "You have plenty of time."

"Not that much," said Bella. "Father had the men load the wagons last night. He expects me to be there when the whistle blows, ready to go with the first one out."

Bella's father had kept his promise. He had found work for her at the mill, if not actually inside it. She had always been mathematically quick, able to figure in her head faster than most people could on paper. It fell to Bella to tally the running board feet of lumber as it was off-loaded from the mill wagons to the flatcars strung along the spur line. A condition of her job was that she neither expect nor receive any special consideration. Her father had told her flatly that he expected her to put in a fair day's work for a fair day's pay, just as he did from everyone else who worked for him. Charlotte knew that David had had reservations. It pleased her as much as it did him that he found Bella to be his best "tallyman" yet.

The man at the door was Peter Hall. "I came by to thank you," he said.

Charlotte nodded. "You really shouldn't be up and about yet," she said. "Another day or two in bed wouldn't have hurt."

He dismissed this with a grin. "I feel just fine, Dr. Ross. Besides, I can't just lay off work as I please."

David had told Charlotte that Peter Hall sent most of his pay packet each month to his family. "Down home," as he would put it, thought Charlotte, on Cape Breton Island. She studied his face. He had an egg over one eye as big as a crow's, as black-and-blue as its shiny ruff. "You should have a cold compress on that eye," she said.

He flushed. "It's not much to worry about." Charlotte's awareness of his injured face made him uncomfortable. "It was a doorknob." The lame lie danced in Peter Hall's eyes. "I bumped into a doorknob." Emboldened, the lie did a pirouette. "Back at the boarding house."

Charlotte tried not to smile. She had heard from Minnie Monilaws, the postmistress, of a knock-down, drag-out fist fight at the Whitemouth House. It had started over something a woodcutter had said to Peter Hall about a woman visitor to his room at the boarding house. The husky young Cape Breton Islander had left the woodcutter bloody and bowed on the sawdust floor of the saloon.

"I was told the circumstances of your accident," said Charlotte, choosing her words carefully. "I hoped your injuries weren't too serious."

Peter Hall hadn't anticipated Charlotte's having heard. His face reddened.

"Opposed as I am to violence, thank you for your gallantry. I daresay that doorknob will think twice," she added drily, "before it opens its mouth again."

A shy smile crept over Peter Hall's bruised face. "You can be sure of that, Dr. Ross. For as long as I'm here in Whitemouth."

Over the next while, Charlotte had time for little else than settling in with her family and preparing for the new baby. There were any number of things to deal with in their new surroundings. From Dr. William Hingston and at medical school, Charlotte had been taught the controversial theories of an Englishman named Edwin Chadwick. Born into a Lancashire farm family, he contended that the best way to deal with disease was to avoid it as much as possible through cleanliness. Although there were many sceptics, Charlotte was not one of them. She was greatly concerned by the threat to her family, to the children especially, of contagious diseases.

It was tiresome work hauling water up from the river on the horse-drawn stone boat and ladling it from barrels into buckets. Despite this, Charlotte and her daughters kept enough water on hand to scrub down the house regularly and to do the wash in two separate tubs. One was used only for clothing and bedsheets. The other was reserved for table linens, kitchen china and cutlery. Most of the money was kept in the safe in David's office at the mill. The little that came into the house was sterilized. Coins were cleansed in boiling water. Paper money was pressed with sadirons heated on top of the cookstove.

It troubled Charlotte when her husband rested the soiled sleeves of the workshirt he was wearing on her boiled and crisply laundered white tablecloths. She asked the mill carpenter to cut two pieces of wood like small bread boards. At supper one evening she wordlessly placed these under his elbows. Whenever David forgot to change into a clean shirt before he sat down at the table, Charlotte brought out the boards. After about a week, David stopped forgetting and the boards disappeared into the woodstove.

Almost from the day that she arrived in Whitemouth, Charlotte began working on two building projects. The first was for a school, the other a church. The school came first. On Sundays the log house on the hill became a Sunday school. Charlotte taught her own two small children and the handful of others who lived close enough to walk or come by horseback. In the evening the house became a place of worship. Preachers passing through were invited to sit down with the family to Sunday dinner. After the sterling serving dishes, fine china and damask table cloth were cleared away, the refectory table and chairs were set back against the log walls. The front door was opened to anyone who cared to enter. The dinner guest, whatever religion he happened to be, was invited to preach. Most of the families who came for evening service came back every Sunday. Whatever voice God happened to be using that week, the Rosses and their neighbours wanted to hear what He had to say.

Hales had turned six in May. He and three of his sisters were school-age. Charlotte discussed this with her husband. The mill was doing even better than David had expected. He agreed to donate the land, the lumber and the hardware, and to bring in a teacher. The school would be built by volunteers. Most had children of their own and were planning to move their families soon to Whitemouth. Almost every week marked the arrival of one or two more. Sometimes they came with their belongings by train from Winnipeg. More often they came by oxcart.

One night early in August, when God's lantern hung amid the uprights and crosspieces of the skeletal schoolhouse, Charlotte took down David's lap desk. She began a letter to her sister-in-law in Winnipeg. After the customary enquiries into Caroline's and William's well-being, she asked Caroline if she would help find a teacher who was willing to move to Whitemouth.

A little more than a week later, Charlotte delivered herself of a son. She was assisted by Bella, who had attended enough births with her mother to qualify as a midwife. While Bella changed the bedclothes, Kate helped her mother gown herself and the baby in nightdresses that Charlotte had sewn with scalloped necklines and wrists of goffered lace.

Min and her younger sister and brother had been sent off to the mill to get their father. They heard them at the front door. Kate took a final hurried brush through her mother's hair while Bella plumped the pillows behind her. David and the children appeared in the doorway. All but Hales, who had ridden on his father's shoulders, were breathless.

"Come in," said Charlotte.

The children ran to her bedside, fussing over the baby.

"Be careful with him," Charlotte cautioned. "He's very new."

"Are you both all right?" asked David, still standing in the doorway.

Charlotte nodded. "The child is sound and I am just a little tired."

David acknowledged this with a smile. He went to his wife and embraced her. Then he carefully took their baby and stood with him. "Joseph Whitehead Ross," he said, trying out the name, deciding it fit. "Your father will like that."

Before the end of the month, Charlotte received a letter from Caroline. Charlotte was well recovered from giving birth. She drove into Whitemouth to pick up the mail. Her sister-in-law's letter had been written on the same day that she had received word from Charlotte about the birth of her son. It was brimming with congratulations and her own good news of the same sort. Her prayers had been answered. She and William were to become parents again in December. She could scarcely wait. The new baby would fill the painful void left in their lives by the death of Ethel Maud. She had already begun work on an elaborate layette.

The letter left Charlotte just a little breathless. She smiled at the page, amused by Caroline's scrawled rush of words. She had been reading as she walked from the post office to the hitching rail out front. Charlotte untethered the horses and climbed into the driver's seat, tying back the reins. She had always found it awkward to try to drive a two-horse team and read at the same time. On Whitemouth's corduroy roads, built to keep spring thaws from turning them into quagmires, it was impossible. Carriages seemed to leap from log to log.

While her team switched tails and nuzzled the tall grass at the side of the road, Charlotte returned to Caroline's letter. James McKay's daughter, Jane Dallas, was to be married at St. Mary's Cathedral the last weekend in August. Her betrothed was a young French lawyer from Normandy named Louis Gagnon. Charlotte reflected that it sounded like a good marriage. Harriett would be pleased. Caroline had found a teacher for the school in Whitemouth. The young woman's name was Sarah Ayr. She was a recent teaching graduate. Caroline listed her references.

Miss Ayr sounded just fine to Charlotte. The schoolhouse was almost finished. The start of the fall term was just a week or so off. They had been fortunate to find a qualified teacher. All that remained was to talk with Mrs. Enright. Although Mrs. Enright didn't know it yet, Sarah Ayr was about to become the first young working woman at her working man's boarding house. Charlotte had gotten to know Mrs. Enright over her week of making house calls on Peter Hall. She was confident that she could persuade her to accept Sarah Ayr as a house guest. Charlotte did not doubt that she would be assigned a room as close as possible to the rigidly proper landlady's own.

Charlotte untied the reins and released the hand brake by her side. The team was anxious to go. When she clucked her tongue the phaeton moved off at a good clip, jolting over the roadbed of moss-covered logs. Alexander and Bryce bragged that their millinery manager had come to Winnipeg by way of some of the best import houses in New York, Chicago and Toronto. She had assured Charlotte that the veiled silk hat with the rolled brim was *de rigueur* for fashionable country living. Charlotte kept a hand clamped down on her hat. In all Miss Beswetherick's travels, Charlotte thought ruefully, she obviously had never heard of corduroy roads.

Charlotte stopped first at the boarding house. She had little difficulty convincing Mrs. Enright that she should provide the school teacher with a place to stay. Over a cup of tea, Charlotte suggested that the young woman would be good company – a pleasant relief from the platoon of men who trooped through the house and formed up in the dining room at mealtimes. She spoke of Mrs. Enright's contribution to the community in assisting with the establishment of the new school. This was important now, Charlotte told her, to the handful of school-age children already in and around Whitemouth. It would be even more so by spring, when the railway west to Winnipeg would be completed from Prince Arthur's Landing, on Lake Superior. Homesteaders were expected to begin arriving by the carload.

Finally, Charlotte pressed, who better to chaperone an innocent and inexperienced young woman than Mrs. Enright herself? Where would she be safer than here? By the time they had finished tea, Mrs. Enright was showing Charlotte the very room for her new boarder. She would pack the two men who now occupied it off to another room on the second floor. Next to her own, she assured Charlotte, this was the brightest and most comfortable bedroom in the house.

Charlotte suppressed a smile. It was also, as she had assumed it would be, right next door to Mrs. Enright's own.

Charlotte's next stop was the railway station. Her team clip-clopped along in close rhythm. The horses were glad to be off once again after a bored snuffle at brown grass, and switching at flies outside Mrs. Enright's. Charlotte checked her watch. She was to catch the train that ran between Winnipeg and Rat Portage to look in on a convalescing accident patient at Cross Lake. The train was due to arrive in Whitemouth at noon. She was in good time.

A week earlier, a young cook's helper had split open his foot chopping firewood at Michael Haney's headquarters, just east of Cross Lake. Hugh Mann was seventeen. His older brother, Donald, had been a foreman under Charlotte's father and had stayed on under Haney. The boy was lucky. The cook had had previous experience with axe cuts, which were common in bush camps. He fashioned a crude tourniquet from a sugar bag and a stick of kindling. The injured youth was wrapped in a bunkhouse blanket and loaded onto a handcar.

Four brawny sectionmen shoved off with him. Donald sat with his brother's head cradled in his arms and an eye on the bandaged foot. Near the end of the run to Whitemouth, he saw his brother's lifeblood stippling the snakes and ladders of rails

204

and ties. Donald panicked. He gave the tourniquet a sharp twist that made his brother cry out. The four workmen, already humping over the pump handles as fast as they could, pumped even harder.

They arrived shouting. The leathers of the brake shoes smoking. One of the pumpers standing hard on the pedal. Donald and the others jumping to the roadbed before the full stop. Tying the corners of the blanket to two saplings to make a litter. David running from the mill. Discarding the slipped tourniquet. Feeling for the artery with his fingers. Pressing on it. Jogging along beside the makeshift stretcher. Heading for the house, so damn far and uphill all the way. And then there. Charlotte at the window; at the door; at the boy's side, taking charge. Neither a man nor a woman, but a doctor doing what she was trained to do. Thank God.

CHAPTER ❦ THIRTEEN

Whitemouth, Fall, 1881

CROSS LAKE was about the same distance again as Whitemouth was from Winnipeg. It cost three dollars return to ride the sixty-five miles or so farther east.

Charlotte took the money from her handbag. She was holding the bills, ready to pay her fare, as the train pulled away from the station. Before they had covered the short run to the Ross mill, the conductor was standing over her. He swayed back and forth to the train's lateral rhythm, his smile as bright as the polished brass buttons on his blue serge suit. He waved off Charlotte's fare.

"No charge, Dr. Ross," he said. "Glad to have you riding with us." He started towards the two other passengers who had got on at Whitemouth. Both were bush workers, judging from their rough dress, and their skin, leathered by exposure to the weather. He turned back to Charlotte. "Next time we'll stop for you at your husband's mill. It will save you going to Whitemouth. Just ask Mr. Ross to have one of his men flag down the engine driver."

The conductor's refusal to take her fare confused Charlotte. So did his offer to make an unscheduled stop for her. "That's very good of you," she said, "but I really couldn't. It's too much to ask."

"Not at all, Dr. Ross." The conductor touched his fingers to his cap. "We do for those who do for us."

Now Charlotte understood. Her treatment of the millworker's illness and the construction-camp cookie's axe wound had brought other men to her door. Although it hadn't occurred to her until now, she had been accepted professionally by the region's bush, mill and railway workers. Her practice was strung out along the railway line from Whitemouth to Rat Portage.

Charlotte leaned forward, reflecting on the wraith-like face in the glass of the coach window. The slash and ground cover of the railway right-of-way slipped by unnoticed. She felt a sense of satisfaction that she had never felt before. This part of her new life more than made up for the difficult times. The years of study and separations from her husband and children had been worth it. It did not matter that she had abandoned family, friends and elegant surroundings to this rude life in a log house in the backwoods. Her practice was no longer limited to women and children, and as an *accoucheur*, as it had been in Montreal. Here she would not just be delivering babies, treating women's diseases and disorders, and applying the industrial-accident skills learned at Pennsylvania Hospital to children's skinned knees and bee stings. Here, finally, she had a full practice.

The thought brought a full smile to the face in the coach window. Charlotte recalled William Luxton's editorial, "Women as Physicians." Because she had thought his closing words were so remarkably patronizing, she remembered them well: "Great Britain is thus to have female doctors who, if they confine themselves to treating their own sex, will do a great deal of good service."

Charlotte wondered what Mr. Luxton would say if he knew that the doctor practising in the work camps between Whitemouth and Rat Portage was a woman, that she was on her way at this moment to treat a young accident victim at Cross Lake. This last thought brought her whimsy up short. Of course William Luxton knew. Or if he didn't already know, he soon would. Little went on anywhere in the province that didn't eventually cross his desk for inclusion in his "City and Regional News" columns.

Charlotte knew something else about William Luxton. Both as publisher of *The Daily Free Press* and as a recent member of the Manitoba Legislature, the man was committed to ridding the province of unlicensed medical practitioners. Whatever their claim to legitimacy, Mr. Luxton lumped them together as opportunists and charlatans. He said that they did more harm than good while picking their patients' pockets. As her train pulled into Cross Lake, Charlotte wondered what steps he might one day take against her and with what result.

Charlotte had applied a linseed poultice to Hugh Mann's wound to draw the poison from an infection that had developed. He was alone in the bunkhouse, lying propped up on one elbow when she entered. She saw that the boy's foot was raw where the poultice had been. The wound itself was no longer inflamed. The lips of the deep gash were drawn cleanly together in healing. What puzzled her was the absence of skin. It had been stripped from his ankle down to his toes. Charlotte set her bag on a table by the bed and sat down at the boy's side. She brushed at a fly that had landed on the exposed tissues.

"Who removed the poultice?" she asked. Gingerly, she touched his ankle. "What happened here?"

"I fell asleep," the boy said. "When I woke up, the mice were eating the flax seeds."

Eating his skin, too, Charlotte realized. She patted his shoulder as she got up. She took a tin of zinc oxide salve and a roll of bandage from her bag. While she lightly coated the raw tissues, Charlotte realized that she was learning some of the special circumstances surrounding her new practice. Like this one, she told herself wryly. She knew now never to apply a linseed poultice to anyone who might be accessible in their sleep to foraging mice. There were other, more serious, difficulties that she wished were as easy to avoid as this one was. She was concerned about never having access to a second opinion. There was no other doctor to confirm or disagree with her diagnosis or prescribed treatment and to suggest alternatives. It made her own decisions mock infallible, until it was perhaps too late to change them. Her other major problem was the absence of a nearby hospital or any facility more antiseptic and better equipped than the spare bedroom she used as an office. The closest was the modest hospital, the original cabin with a house built onto it, run by the Grey Nuns in St. Boniface.

Charlotte looped the fresh bandage several times around her young patient's foot, loosely enough to let the healing air circulate. She smoothly knotted the bandage, then stepped back to appraise her work.

"There!" she said, satisfied. "Except for the damage done by the mice, your wound is clean and healing well."

Charlotte had been practising medicine for six years. Despite the problems of isolation, she felt that only since coming to Whitemouth had she found the challenge and fulfillment whose promise had taken her to Philadelphia.

On the last Saturday in September, Charlotte's father arrived at the Ross mill. He was travelling with Sir Charles Tupper and a government party aboard the minister of railways' special train. They had spent the previous day in Brandon, rolling west from Winnipeg over newly laid track that was not yet open to the public.

In Brandon, Charlotte's older brother had bought the first land to be sold by the Canadian Pacific from the vast acreage it had been granted along its right-of-way west. He and Sir Charles had met in the Pullman palace car that served both as a ministerial residence and an office on rails. Sir Charles had acted for the Land Department of the railway. The sale to Charles was the first step in the government's plan to turn the prairies into farmland, and populate the West. The Land Department's Contract No. 1 covered a square mile of fertile grassland in the valley of the Assiniboine River. The deal had been sealed with a handshake.

Sir Charles's train, with the government party and Charlotte's father on board, had made the return run to Winnipeg late that night. On the first call to breakfast it had left for Selkirk, the Ross mill at Whitemouth, Cross Lake and Rat Portage.

Charlotte and her father were standing by the train. They were waiting for Sir Charles to emerge.

"Charles is calling his place Broadline Farm," said Joseph. "He's putting it in wheat and oats the first year. He's also started a dairy herd with blood cattle that he's brought in from Oshawa."

Charlotte was about to ask after Hanna and the children when Sir Charles stepped down from his private railway car. She had always thought the man's career to be fascinating. He had left a successful medical practice to enter politics and be elected premier of Nova Scotia. With Sir John A. Macdonald, Sir Charles had been one of the principal architects of Confederation fourteen years earlier. He was also the founding president of the Canadian Medical Association. Dr. William Hingston had been founding secretary.

Joseph introduced Sir Charles to Charlotte.

"We have a mutual friend in Montreal," said the railways minister. "He asks that I convey his respects and good wishes. As the fortunate courier, I beg to add my own to those of Dr. Hingston."

Charlotte smiled acknowledgement. Sir Charles was about a half-dozen years shy of her father's sixty-six. She judged that he had the sense of self of a skilled surgeon and the silver tongue of a career politician.

"I have not seen Dr. Hingston since leaving Montreal. That was four years ago this past August. I assume he is well?"

"He is."

"And his wife, Margaret Josephine?"

"I am pleased to say equally so."

"He is an old and valued friend. He sends me the bulletins issued by the Canadian Medical Association. Two or three times a year," she laughed, "in large bundles. They are a great help to me in keeping current with my profession."

"Dr. Hingston spoke very highly of you, but not without some concern. He expressed distress that you might still be practising unlicensed." Sir Charles frowned his disapproval. "The time for that is past. We can purge ourselves of quackery only through strict enforcement of the law. Quite frankly, dear lady, I must echo Dr. Hingston's distress with anyone, no matter how well qualified, who defies it."

Charlotte's words came measured. "Like other women, I was obliged to go elsewhere to study medicine. The country that refused to school me should not demand that I return to school here to be qualified. My doctorate is my licence."

Sir Charles was gruffly sympathetic. "There is change in the wind."

"It comes too late for some of us."

"This past summer, a special course of studies was established in Kingston, Ontario, for women. It's offered by Queen's University."

"I do not intend to return to the classroom to qualify myself to practise," said Charlotte. "For one thing, I am thirty-seven years this past summer." She smiled faintly. "A trifle mature for a schoolgirl. For another, my life is too full to allow it. I have a husband, four daughters between the ages of eight and nineteen, a six-year-old son, and a six-week-old infant. I would be hard-pressed to find time for Kingston."

At the beginning of their conversation, Charlotte's father and the others had gone with David to look at his mill. As they reappeared down the track, Sir Charles bowed to Charlotte. "It has been a pleasure, Dr. Ross. I will extend your good wishes to Dr. Hingston and his wife on my return to Montreal."

On the first Monday in December, Charlotte took the train to Winnipeg. Caroline was expecting momentarily. Charlotte spent the waiting days visiting friends that she had made during the time she had lived in the house on Dagmar Street. She also helped William move his drugstore to the new Duffin Building at Main and Bannatyne streets. On Sunday, Charlotte delivered her sister-in-law of a son, William Jr.

The afternoon before her return to Whitemouth, Charlotte dropped in on her brother at his new location. She nodded to him from behind two waiting customers while he served another. The business, Caroline had told her, was continuing to do even better than they had anticipated. William's success was due partly to the attractive and often unusual items with which he stocked his shelves. For the Christmas opening of his new store he had brought in ornaments and gift miniatures of straw. Artfully woven from dried grasses, they were imported from Germany.

Charlotte spoke on the heels of the last departing customer.

"Mr. Luxton in his newspaper describes your store as a fairy bower."

William nodded. He was silent while his sister chose a straw miniature for each of the children. As she handed them across the counter, his frown told her that something was troubling him.

"You look glum for a proud new father," she said. "What's wrong?"

William scowled. "Your medical practice."

Charlotte studied him a moment. "I don't understand."

"You've upset some members of the medical profession in Winnipeg. Your activities here haven't gone unnoticed, even though you may have thought they did."

"What you're saying is that I've ruffled a few cock feathers."

William nodded. "You have. Quite a few."

"More to the point, I've taken money out of their pockets."

"That, too. It's a fact of life."

"It's an unfair one. Women who want a woman doctor should have the choice. It shouldn't be just a case of male pride and money. You know yourself that I've never sought out patients or pressed for fees."

William knew this was true. Salaried workers and their families, and those who charged for goods or services, paid Charlotte in cash, her bill based on how well off they were. Most of the homesteaders gave her freshly caught sturgeon, game, farm produce, or wild berry preserves. More often than not, especially among new arrivals, Charlotte provided medical care without charge. Nevertheless, her practice had cost William professional friends and prescription referrals.

"It has become an issue," he said. "Particularly because of my position with the Pharmaceutical Association."

"I'm sorry."

William saw his sister's apology for what it was. Regret, not capitulation. He knew it would never be that. "I hear that not many people from Whitemouth on up the line are coming to Winnipeg for treatment any more. You must be keeping busy."

Charlotte smiled. "Happily so."

William grunted. "I also hear you've been treating Indians."

This surprised Charlotte. She had not realized that her small and isolated practice was attracting so much attention. "Father Lacombe sent me my first Indian patient. She was a young Saulteaux woman. Her husband brought her from Fort Alexander. It took them three days by canoe, but she didn't care. She said she couldn't wait for the next visit by the treaty doctor, whenever that would be. She said that when he did come, he treated them like cattle. Men and women were told to undress and were examined in the same room. Father Lacombe was as shocked as I was."

Father Lacombe was a frequent after-dinner preacher at the Ross house. His Grace Archbishop Alexandre Taché had removed him from St. Mary's Cathedral and made him the Canadian Pacific Railway chaplain. Father Lacombe's mission was to bring a little godliness to the generally drunken and debauched railway-construction workers. His church was a boxcar at any of the thirty camps strung out between St. Boniface and Eagle River, well into northwestern Ontario.

Charlotte enjoyed the priest's visits. It gave her the opportunity to resurrect the school French that had won her the medal at the Convent of the Sacred Heart. Father Lacombe appreciated the conversation, the comfortable surroundings and the home-cooked dinners.

Charlotte would have liked to spend a few more days in Winnipeg. Even though she had finished her Christmas shopping, she was enjoying her stay with William, Caroline and the baby. But David had asked that she be back by the following Sunday. He was leaving the day after that to set up a winter bush camp northeast of Whitemouth. Burdened with Christmas gifts, Charlotte took the train from Winnipeg on Saturday morning.

David left with his foreman and their Indian guide early Monday. He promised to be back in six days for Christmas, their first in Whitemouth.

David's second night out, Charlotte was startled awake by a loud pounding at the door.

"Mother?" Bella had heard it, too. She was standing barefoot in her nightdress at the doorway to her mother's bedroom, huddled by the door; they were joined within the moment by her sister Kate.

Again, "Mother?" – tremulously.

Charlotte got up and went to the bedroom closet. She took down her night robe and wrapped it around her. She lighted a coal-oil lamp and a lantern, motioning to her two daughters to be quiet, gesturing to them to look to their two younger sisters and Hales. These three had now trailed sleepy-eyed from their bedrooms. Charlotte walked with the lantern to the door, cocking her head to listen, taking a step back, startled, as the pounding resumed.

"There's a man badly wounded!" a voice shouted. "Maybe dying!"

Charlotte glanced at her three older daughters. She had noticed how some of the men looked at them. She crossed the floor to the pegged gun rack on the far wall. David had taken the newer and more rapid firing Winchester 73. He had left behind the rifle he had brought west with him, a Spencer seven-shot repeater. The forerunner to the Winchester, it was slower and heavier, but no less reliable.

Charlotte took down the rifle and thumbed back the mule-ear hammer that had to be cocked by hand after each shot. This gun was kept loaded. There were sometimes black bear about, which could usually be frightened off with a warning shot. Wolves had been known to sink their teeth into pigs' ears and drag them off into the surrounding bush.

Charlotte walked to the front door and levelled the Spencer waist-high. "I have a loaded rifle pointed at this door," she called out in a calm voice. "I promise I'll shoot the first man who comes through it!"

The pounding stopped. She could hear voices, but not what was being said.

"We've a friend who's near dead!" someone finally shouted.

"He needs a doctor!"

Charlotte considered this a moment. "Have you got him with you?"

"He's hurt too bad! He's back at the CP Hotel!"

Charlotte looked at her children. Bella had picked up the baby. Startled from his sleep by the loud voices, he had awakened, crying. Bella was standing at the doorway to his bedroom with him cradled in her arms. She was making soothing and hushing sounds. Kate and Min stood frightened but steadfast with Carrie and Hales, prepared to defend the two younger ones from whatever devils threatened beyond the door. Charlotte gave them a nod of reassurance that she herself did not feel. As their mother, she could not risk a hair on their heads. As a doctor, she could not refuse medical aid to a seriously injured, perhaps dying, man. She thought of a possible solution and seized upon it. "If what you say is true," she called out, "send for Peter Hall."

Whenever David was away, Charlotte knew that the young millworker from Cape Breton Island would be somewhere close by. On the morning that he had shown up at her door with a black eye, he had appointed himself her protector. Most of the men in and around Whitemouth knew each other by name. The men outside her door would know in which of the town's three hotels they would find Peter Hall. Charlotte cocked her head close to the bolted and barred door, trying to catch what was being said on the other side.

"All right!" the man who had done most of the talking

shouted. "We'll go find Hall!"

Charlotte pressed closer to the door.

"It's a far piece," someone said. "What if we don't make it back in time?"

"If we don't, we don't," she heard the reply. "We can't just bust in and haul her back with us."

Charlotte had heard enough. She was reasonably sure that the men were not just trying to gain entry to the house. "Wait!" she called out. She carefully uncocked the Spencer and leaned it against the wall. She faced the children. "Don't worry," she said. "It's all right. Go back to bed, all of you." She waited until they were in their rooms. Then she lifted the iron bar from the brackets that barred the door, and drew back the bolt. She opened the door a slit and shone her lantern on the three men standing in the fresh December snow. She thought two of them looked familiar. Reassured, she opened the door wide. "What happened?" she asked.

"There was a fight in the bar. Someone pulled a knife. Our friend's cut real bad. The bleeding won't stop."

Charlotte gave the man the lantern. "There's a horse and sleigh in the barn," she said. "Hitch up. I'll be ready when you are." She closed the door and walked quickly to her room. Bella met her at the entrance with the lamp.

"I'll want my bag," Charlotte said, shrugging off her night robe as she spoke. She took warm underclothing from her bureau drawer and crossed to the closet. "When I'm gone bolt and bar the door. The rifle's leaning against the wall beside it. You know how to cock and use it, if you need to." She dressed quickly. "I'm counting on you to see that no harm comes to yourself or the other children. Do you understand?"

Bella nodded. She was wide-eyed, not from her mother's matter-of-fact instructions, but from the tumble of events that had begun with the pounding at the door. "I'll get your bag," she said.

"I'll need needle and thread," Charlotte called after her. "You'll find both in my sewing basket. Choose a good-sized needle and coarse black silk."

The needle and thread were for suturing. Charlotte preferred a quality silk, although she knew that some saddleback surgeons simply used a hair plucked from their horse's tail.

Charlotte arrived at the front door at the same time as the horse and sleigh. Two of the three men sat in front, one holding the reins. The third took Charlotte's bag and gave her a hand up onto the seat beside him. She was scarcely settled when the driver let out a shout and laid the reins across the horse's flanks. With a sudden jerk they were off for Whitemouth.

When they pulled up in front of the Canadian Pacific Hotel, a handful of men were standing in the yellow wedge of light at the half-open door. They were drinking from a common bottle, passing it unsteadily from one to another. They were either oblivious to the cold, Charlotte decided, or, what was more likely, immune to it. A boisterous cheer went up as she stepped down from the sleigh. The man who had been driving tied the reins to the hitching rail. The other two cleared a path for her into the hotel.

A group of men standing by the bar parted as Charlotte's escort hurried her towards them, calling out to make way. At their centre the wounded man sat at a card table. The saloonkeeper, his white apron stained dark red, was standing over him. He was holding a dishtowel to the man's neck. Both the cloth and the fingers that held it were caked with blood.

Dark red and caked, Charlotte saw with some relief. She set her bag down on the table and flipped open its metal snaps. Bright red blood, pumped fresh from the heart, would have meant an artery. The man likely would have been dead by now. His condition was still serious. A slashed jugular, Charlotte thought, from the look of it.

"I've kept a towel pressed tight against his neck," said the saloonkeeper.

"You did the right thing," said Charlotte. "You probably saved his life."

The man looked pleased with himself.

"I'll need someone to hold a lamp close. A basin of hot water. Some clean towels."

Charlotte took over from the saloonkeeper. She kept the crusted towel pressed against the wound. One of the men watching took down a reflector lamp and stood beside her. Charlotte bent and looked into the wounded man's eyes. He was not going into severe shock, as she expected. "How do you feel?"

222

"I'm all right. I'm still here."

"Good."

"I need some whiskey."

"No you don't."

The saloonkeeper brought a basin of hot water and some towels. Charlotte gently sponged the man's neck. The cut was clean, but deep. The knife had slashed through the layered tissues and across the membranous wall of the external jugular.

Thank God the man is in his prime, thought Charlotte, and apparently as healthy as a horse. She took a bottle of diluted carbolic acid and a cloth from her bag. She uncorked the bottle and soaked the cloth and her hands. She gently dabbed at the wound, letting the antiseptic solution run over and into it. The man sat in stoic silence.

"Are you a woodsman?" asked Charlotte. She put the bottle back in her bag and took out a needle and thread.

"I am."

"I thought as much."

Charlotte motioned the man with the lamp to hold it higher. She threaded the needle. Then she raised the lamp's glass chimney and sterilized it over the flame. "This will hurt," she said. She gingerly exposed the cut in the vein. She turned to the man with the lamp. "Come closer." She waited until the full light from the lamp's tin reflector played on the wound. Then she began stitching.

The light from the lamp wavered. Charlotte shot a look at the man holding it. "Steady," she said.

She finished suturing the vein and cut the thread. The bleeding had almost stopped. She drew together the open wound in the man's neck. His skin was weathered to the colour and toughness of leather. The oozing blood made her fingers and the needle slippery. Charlotte glanced around her. On a nearby table lay some scattered poker chips. She asked for one. It made a thimble. She used it to push the needle through the skin until the wound was sutured.

Throughout, the woodsman sat silent and practically un-moving. Both hands gripped his thighs. Sometimes Charlotte saw his eyes squeeze shut, and his mouth become a hard line. That was all. She cut the thread with her scissors. "It's done." She placed a hand on his shoulder. "You can have a whiskey now. You've earned it."

David arrived back home, as he had promised he would, on Christmas Eve. Because it was their first Christmas in their new home, Charlotte wanted it to be special. She knew it could not be like the well-remembered ones in Clinton, with all the shops as gay as gift wrap and the continuous comings and goings at her father's house. Still, she was determined to do her best. Fresh eggs, cream and butter from their own hens and cow had gone into the cookies and shortbreads. Instead of the spiced shoulder of beef, bagged in white linen, that had always been a part of their Christmas, a saddle of venison hung from the ceiling of the root cellar. In place of the usual barrel of fresh oysters, there were steaks cut from sturgeon gaffed in the whitewater at the foot of

Whitemouth Falls. Charlotte's father had arrived the day before David did. His contribution, which he had brought with him from back east, was a wheel of well-aged white Cheddar cheese.

On Christmas Day, Charlotte was busy dividing the dinner chores among herself and her three older daughters when David came into the kitchen. He had a frown on his face. "There is a man at the door," he said. "He has heard that we welcome preachers and asks permission to hold a service."

While he had never actually said as much, Charlotte knew that David did not fully approve of this. He had a strong sense of family privacy and an unshakeable faith as a Presbyterian. "We have opened our doors to Anglicans, Methodists and Roman Catholics, as well as our own," he said. "Now we have a man of no particular religious stripe, an evangelist, apparently, who calls himself Father Christmas."

"Does he look like Father Christmas?" asked Charlotte. David missed the veiled smile. "Well, I suppose he does," he admitted. "At any rate, he has a white beard and wears a red toque."

"Then what better person to welcome into our home on Christmas Day?" asked Charlotte. She slipped an arm through her husband's. "Do ask Father Christmas if he would care to join us for dinner."

CHAPTER ❦ FOURTEEN

Whitemouth, Summer, 1882

*T*HE FAMILY had just eaten breakfast. Charlotte and David lingered over a last few sips of tea. Bella, Kate, Min and Carrie sat waiting for them to finish. Baby Joseph was sprawled in his high chair near his mother. Hales, who would not be seven for another four days, had been permitted to leave the table. He was standing by the kitchen window, looking down on the river and the road that led from the mill.

"Someone's coming," he said.

Bella was up and across the floor before Charlotte could speak. She placed her hands on her brother's shoulders, bending over him to see who it was.

"Bella!" Although it came too late to stop her eldest daughter, Charlotte's commanding tone was not lost on her three younger daughters. They remained fastened to their chairs.

"It's Father Lacombe," said Bella. She walked demurely back to the table and sat down.

"As the eldest, you should set a better example for your brothers and sisters," said her mother.

Charlotte's English Methodist upbringing had been as severe as David's Scottish Presbyterian one. Today would be like every other Sunday. It was a day of self-restraint and rest. Wood had been cut and laid the night before. All that was needed to fire up the cookstove was to light it. By mid-morning Charlotte would be teaching Sunday school for her own small children and the few others who lived nearby. Carrie and Hales would spend the afternoon leafing through picture books of Queen Victoria and the Royal family, and British history. Later there would be a hymn-sing, accompanied on the piano by Charlotte or one of her three older daughters. She had taught them all how to play. In the evening, the preacher who was their guest at dinner would hold a service.

"You may go and welcome Father Lacombe," said Charlotte.

Although Bella managed not to appear unseemly, she was the first up from the table. Charlotte caught the amusement in her husband's eyes. She shook her head and reached for the baby. Joseph was mouthing a small tray. Just the right size and fashioned from thin silver, its most practical use was as a teething aid. Charlotte had yet to meet anyone from Whitemouth to Rat Portage who carried a calling card.

Father Lacombe was in high spirits. In just a few days, track-laying between the northwest shores of Lake Superior and Winnipeg would be completed. "I'm on my way home," he told the Rosses. "To Fort Calgary and the Bow River country."

Charlotte knew that the priest's mission had been a hard one. A few months earlier he had fallen seriously ill. She had taken him into her home and treated him for pleurisy. Throughout the winter, whatever the weather, he had been making the rounds of the railway-construction camps by handcar. The long hours and exposure to the elements had finally caught up with him. During a spell of low spirits and high fever, Father Lacombe had told Charlotte that Rat Portage and Eagle River were his Sodom and Gomorrah.

The horse and buggy he was driving, camp gear to take him west, and a new saddle, had come as a complete surprise. They were a going-away gift. Just about everyone in the camps had chipped in to buy them for him.

"You must have reached a few hearts," said Charlotte. "More than you knew."

The priest nodded. "Hopefully a few souls, too," he said.

Father Lacombe did not have time to take tea with Charlotte and her family. He had his final report to make that evening to Archbishop Taché, at St. Boniface Cathedral. He vaulted up into the driver's seat. Father Lacombe showed off his new buggy a little, bringing it about in a tight wheel in front of the family. He responded to their goodbyes with a waved blessing. Then he started off at a comfortable trot down the short road to the Whitemouth River and the longer one to the Bow.

On the first Wednesday in July, the Countess of Dufferin struck out for Prince Arthur's Landing on the shores of Thunder Bay. It arrived at midnight. It began its return trip that same afternoon. Aboard the train were the first homesteaders to ship by steamer from Toronto to The Lakehead and travel west by Canadian Pacific. Some were families from Ontario and Quebec. Most were emigrants from Europe.

Charlotte's practice took a new turn. The railway-construction gangs had left Manitoba. They were laying track across the prairies of the North-West Territories towards Pile of Bones and Fort Calgary. With the coming of the homesteaders, Charlotte became a family doctor.

Sometimes she drove the phaeton on her house calls. Where there were no roads, which was usually the case, she went by horseback. Where there were not even saddle-horse trails, she took the train. It stopped for her by the mill. It made another unscheduled stop wherever the engine driver saw someone sitting in a wagon by the track. This happened sometimes by a partly cleared field, often by a set of ruts. Starting at trackside, these ruts would wander haphazardly off into the bush, stumbling finally on the unseen shack that was a homestead family's first house.

On the train's return run, the engine driver stopped for Charlotte where he had dropped her. If she wasn't there, he gave a series of hurry-up hoots on his steam whistle. When Charlotte arrived she acknowledged his stopping with a wave. Then she boarded one of the immigrant coaches with board seats that served as passenger cars between Winnipeg and The Lakehead. In an emergency, when she couldn't wait for a train, Charlotte rode a handcar pumped by any four sectionmen that she could press into service.

Early in August, the station at Cross Lake telegraphed Whitemouth, reporting that a homesteader clearing his land had been caught by a falling tree. The lower part of his leg was crushed. The Whitemouth telegrapher acknowledged the message on his Morse key. He sent a sectionman to the Ross house. When Charlotte arrived, she found only the telegrapher, one other sectionman and the agent, a young man named William Barton, at the station. The telegrapher could not leave his key. Charlotte set out by handcar with the agent and the two sectionmen pumping.

They had not gone far before Charlotte grew impatient with the slow time that only three pairs of hands could make. She stood in with the station agent. William Barton opened his mouth to protest. He bit his tongue when he saw the determined look on Charlotte's face. The two sectionmen exchanged delighted grins.

It was a hot day, even for mid-summer in Manitoba. As she pumped, Charlotte reflected that, while gentlemen were said to perspire and ladies to blush, the four of them were plain sweating.

As the handcar's wheels clicked away the distance between Whitemouth and the Ross mill, her wet hands threatened to slip from the pump handle. She waited for the upward swing. Then she grabbed at the hem of her skirts, wiping her palms dry on her petticoats.

Charlotte amputated the homesteader's right leg. She took it off just below the knee on the kitchen table of the family's unplaned board cabin. She used a carpenter's handsaw. It was brought to her from where it hung on a nail in the stable by the eldest of the man's eight children. She anaesthetized him by

THE 🌹 IRON 🌹 ROSE

wrapping his face in a towel and dripping chloroform into it from a bottle with a split cork. Then she showed the man's wife how to continue the dripping so that he would remain unconscious.

Charlotte began by pulling the skin upwards, towards the thigh. She cut with her scalpel through the drawn skin, the tissues and sinews. Then she sawed through the bone. The scalpel and the rest of her surgical instruments had been wrapped in layers of newspaper and baked sterile in her cookstove at home. They were kept germ-free in their newsprint cocoons until they were needed. She had sterilized the handsaw in a strong wash of carbolic acid. Charlotte drew the skin of the man's leg down over the cauterized stump. She sutured it with her sewing needle and silk thread. Then she took the towel from his face and brought him back to consciousness.

Charlotte sat up with the man and his wife through the night. A home-made lamp burned on the rough pine table at his bedside. The lamp was a squat bottle filled with coal oil. A wick had been pushed through a hole punched in its cap. A pin was used to raise or lower the flame. The man's wife had lit it with a blind match, which meant that there was no sulphur eye to the long, thin stick. It was used to transfer flame from stove to lamp and back again. In this way, a box of matches bought at the store lasted several months.

When day broke, the homesteader's eldest son hitched up the wagon to drive Charlotte to trackside. Charlotte guessed that the boy was barely into his teens, but he was aged beyond his years. In the stable, she told him that he would have to be even more responsible now. She showed him how to carve a peg leg from the length of white pine that he brought from the wood-shed. When his father was well-enough healed, the peg leg could be fitted with leather straps to the stump of his leg. Charlotte promised to drop by each week over the next while.

She sat in silence as the old wagon creaked and groaned over the parallel ruts that sought out the edge of the forest. The mother had told her that they had emigrated from Germany the previous spring. Most of the homesteaders were from Germany. Or Austria. Or Russia. They had fled military press gangs and traded what little they had for even less. The difference, the mother had been quick to point out, was that here there was a promise for the future.

Charlotte glanced at the boy seated next to her in the driver's box. He wore a clean shirt that had been cut and sewn from a flour sack. A house of the sort they had just left could be built for seventy-five cents – the cost of glass for the windows, nails and unplaned boards. Clay mixed with straw and molded over ash poles for strength had made a chimney. Dried, then heat-fired, it became a kind of brick. In three years, for ten dollars, the family would get ritle to 160 acres. Providing, thought Charlotte, that a one-legged man, his wife and a boy could make it all work for a family of ten.

Charlotte did not have the lengthy wait at trackside for the regular passenger train between Fort William and Winnipeg. Just minutes after she and the boy pulled up in the farm wagon, a work train stopped for her. It was on its way from Rat Portage to the Ross mill to take on several carloads of railway ties. Charlotte rode in the cab with the stoker and the engine driver. Both lived in Whitemouth at Mrs. Enright's boarding house.

As the train lurched into motion, Charlotte watched the boy start the wagon back to the homestead. She was not really seeing him. Her mind was on an early visit to Winnipeg. In May her husband's cousin, Donald Ross Dingwall, had closed down a jewellery store he had bought in Port Hope, Ontario, and had come west with his wife, Margaret. He had located on Main Street, just a block or so north of William's drugstore. Charlotte was looking forward to visiting the new shop. Her penchant for pretty things had not been diminished by the homely life she led in Whitemouth. If anything, she realized, it had become more pronounced. Charlotte idly noticed that the farm wagon, already lost in her thoughts, had disappeared into the forest. Soon her head was nodding to the metallic lullaby of wheels on rails. The next thing she knew, the engine driver was calling her name. She had not slept since rising with the sun the previous morning, several hours before leaving Whitemouth by handcar. When she looked out from the engine cab, she was surprised to see her husband's mill. It was only then that she realized how very tired she must have been.

By mid-summer, construction of the Canadian Pacific Railway had crossed Manitoba and was pressing into the North-West. While some ballast and grading work was still being done between Fort William and Cross Lake, rails were being laid over the flat run to Fort Calgary as fast as they could be horsed into place. Already change was in the prairie wind. A visit to end of track was made late in August by Sir John Campbell, Marquess of Lorne, who had succeeded Lord Dufferin as governor general. He was accompanied by his wife, Princess Alice. She renamed the old buffalo-killing grounds in honour of her mother, Queen Victoria. Pile of Bones became Regina.

Charlotte was seeking change herself. From her first days in Whitemouth she had been campaigning for vaccination against smallpox. Opposition had been successful in Montreal. Even now, seven years after the anti-vaccination riots, Coderre and his followers managed to keep the immunity program from becoming law. What Charlotte encountered in Whitemouth was a stubborn if good-natured resistance based on hearsay. It was as if Dr. Coderre's shouted protests were being heard in Manitoba, even though they came as just a whisper.

Charlotte was continually frustrated in her attempts to persuade just one of the local people to be the first to be vaccinated. She knew that she had to demonstrate that vaccination was both harmless and practically painless. To do this, she realized that she had to vaccinate one of their own.

Near the end of January, twenty members of a track-grading gang from far up the line rode the train to Winnipeg into Whitemouth. They had packed that morning and fled Rosslyn Camp, eight miles east of Rat Portage. One railway-construction worker had died of smallpox the previous day. A second lay dying in his bunkhouse bed. When the train stopped at

Whitemouth to take on passengers and a load of lumber from the Ross mill, the station agent heard about the outbreak from the conductor. William Barton sent a message to the Ross house. Charlotte caught the next scheduled train east from Winnipeg to Thunder Bay.

She found the camp all but deserted. A cook's helper, who said he could not leave the sick man to freeze to death, had stayed behind. Everyone else had run off to Rat Portage or Winnipeg. The cookie had kept the stove going in the bunkhouse, keeping a cautious distance between himself and the man on the bed. Twice a day he had edged close enough to hand him a cup of hot soup. Since the previous day, he told Charlotte, the man had not been well enough to take the soup. The cookie was glad to see her. He brought the gruel she requested, and more firewood, then left the bunkhouse.

Charlotte knew that there was nothing she could do for the dying man. He brushed away the cup that she put to his lips. When his brow broke out in sweat she stuffed her scarf with snow, knotting each end, to make a cold pack. She held it to his forehead. For the long hours until the setting sun showed orange in the bunkhouse window, she made him as comfortable as she could. She sat by him in silence. When the room began to grow colder, she got up and put another log in the woodstove. When the twilight came to the window, telling her that night was near, it came to the man's eyes as well. For a short time he was rational. Charlotte spoke to him soothingly. She asked him if he believed in God. He said he did. She took both his hands in hers. They prayed together until death and the darkness came.

Charlotte returned home from Rosslyn Camp with the feeling that the smallpox virus had shown uncommon restraint. It had claimed the lives of just two workmen. She hoped that these two deaths might prove enough to prompt someone in Whitemouth to volunteer to be vaccinated. She was disappointed. Two victims as far removed as Rosslyn Camp were not close enough to put the fear of a smallpox epidemic into the people of Whitemouth. Charlotte knew that the virus could travel as fast as a human carrier. She had an uneasy feeling that it was much nearer than anyone realized.

With the hard winter months of February and March behind, Charlotte had more personal things to occupy her thoughts. Foremost among these was Whitemouth's first church wedding. Ross Presbyterian Church had been built by volunteer labour over the previous summer, and was finished in late fall. It was a milled-log building with a small front vestibule, both with vertical-slab roofs as sharply pitched as arrowheads. There were two large windows on each side. Charlotte's husband had donated the land, the lumber, the glass and the hardware. On the first Sunday of each month, it was Ross Presbyterian. On the second it served as Ross Methodist. On the third as Ross Anglican. On the fourth as Ross Roman Catholic. On the first four Sundays, from the family pew that was third from the front on the west side, Charlotte saw little difference from the services that had been held in the house. While the denomination changed from week to week, the face of the congregation remained about the same.

Bella wished to be the first bride to be married in the church that had been named for her family. The man she chose was Fremont Wood, a mining engineer from Detroit City, Michigan. He had visited Whitemouth the previous fall, following the railway and new mines exploration through northwestern Ontario into Manitoba. They had met on a morning in late October.

Bella had been standing by the tracks, pencil and clipboard in hand, tallying the lumber being off-loaded onto a flatcar. The young American engineer had left the post office, where he had gone to mail a letter to a friend back east, and was walking back to his hotel. A roundabout route to the Whitemouth House had brought him by the railway station. The sight of a woman tallying at a flatcar loading caught his eye. He had not noticed immediately how attractive she was. Fremont had never before seen a young lady working at anything other than teaching school or clerking in an office. He had reacted with surprise. Then scepticism. Then amused admiration as he watched her call out and note the board footage by unit and mounting total, as fast as the crew could off-load and stack it.

When the job was finished, he had walked over to Bella with a confident smile and an engaging hello. He had proposed to her less than two months later, while a guest at the Rosses' for Christmas dinner. David had given his consent the following week. The wedding had been set for the second Wednesday in April, three months before Bella's twenty-first birthday.

Charlotte's misgivings over the betrothal were lost on both her eldest daughter and her husband. From the day Fremont and Bella had met, she was concerned that a succession of departures had been made from what was both prudent and socially acceptable. The fact that Fremont had not waited to be properly introduced to her daughter was the first of Charlotte's concerns. More important, she believed that their engagement, like the brief time they had known each other beforehand, had been much too short. It also bothered her that beyond his name, birthplace and the fact that he made his living as a mining engineer, she and David knew practically nothing about the man who was about to become their son-in-law. Finally, although Charlotte understood that her feelings in this case meant little to her headstrong eldest daughter, she had never been all that fond of Fremont Wood. She openly conceded him an abundance of charm. Privately, her character assessment was significantly more frugal.

Charlotte's father arrived in Whitemouth on the day before his granddaughter's wedding. He brought a Norwich canary as a gift for Charlotte. He had bought it on impulse while passing a Main Street shop that specialized in songbirds and japanned brass cages. The proprietor had suggested the Norwich. Nicknamed the "John Bull of canaries," it was bold and stocky, with a commanding song. Its plumage was hot yellow and burnt orange. The proprietor had told Joseph that the breed was a great favourite among fashionable Victorian ladies. Back east and in England, many carried them with them in their lacquered black cages.

Charlotte and her father had not seen each other for some weeks. Both welcomed the opportunity to share an hour or so over afternoon tea. David was down at the mill. Bella and Fremont were off together somewhere. Min, Carrie and Hales were in school. Kate was caring for the baby. Because the house was not large enough to accommodate all of them overnight, Charles and William and their families planned to arrive by train the next morning and return home immediately after the wedding reception.

Charlotte was both pleased and puzzled by her father's gift. She gave it pride of place in the main room, directly in front of the window overlooking the Whitemouth River. Her father watched her.

"I'm glad you like him," he said.

"He's precious!" said Charlotte. "But such a surprise!" She shook her head to show her bewilderment. "A canary, of all things! Whatever prompted you?"

"A talk with William Luxton," said her father. "About cats, oddly enough."

"Cats?"

"Luxton told me someone's having cats shipped out from the East. They're to be sold for one dollar each. As companions."

Charlotte laughed. "I doubt my John Bull would want one."

Her father shrugged. "A cat isn't practical here in

Whitemouth. If a wolf didn't get it, something else would. Being safe in his cage and easy to care for, I thought the canary might be good company."

Charlotte was touched by her father's thoughtfulness. It nonetheless bothered her that he obviously still thought of her as a proper Victorian lady – an eccentric one, unaccountably, who had chosen a log drawingroom. She got up and walked to the cage. "I lead a very full life," she said. "Perhaps something little will satisfy that small part of me that is left to be lonely."

"I have heard how busy you are." Joseph hesitated. "How could I help but hear? You have the respect of every railroader from Whitemouth east to Wabigoon Lake. Every homesteader, too, apparently. I was told the region will soon be overrun with girls named Charlotte and boys named David. All in your honour."

Charlotte did not trust herself to turn and face her father. If this finally was his acknowledgement, after so many years, it threatened to overwhelm her. She remained silent.

Joseph cleared his throat. "I did not approve when you chose to study medicine. I have to admit that I still don't. You made up your mind to do it, with or without my blessing, and you did it well. You did it so well that you've made me very proud."

It was thirteen years since the summer they had quarrelled by the croquet pitch at Glengarry over her resolve to enrol that fall in the Woman's Medical College of Pennsylvania. Charlotte turned and faced her father. She did not trust herself to speak. Joseph extended his arms. It was like a late invitation, awk-

wardly delivered by an embarrassed host. Charlotte accepted it
graciously. She walked smiling into her father's embrace.

"I have something else to tell you," he said.

Charlotte drew back. Her expression was quizzical. She knew
what her father had just finished saying had not been easy for
him. He did not lend words ungrudgingly to his emotions. She
had the feeling that this also was something he had taken pains
to rehearse.

"You must have noticed how often I have been to Montreal
over the past while."

Charlotte nodded. "I know you have business interests there."

"A personal interest, too."

Charlotte abruptly knew what her father was about to say.
She wondered why it hadn't dawned on her sooner. She looked
at once surprised and pleased for him. The quick warmth of her
reaction made him smile.

"I have been seeing Harriett McKay since she moved to
Montreal. We were good friends before she left Winnipeg. She
has agreed to be my wife."

Charlotte impulsively took both her father's hands in hers.
"When? Where?"

"Saturday. My train arrives in London that morning. Harriett
will leave Montreal on Friday and meet me there. I've arranged
for a simple ceremony. Just the reverend and the required two
witnesses."

Charlotte looked her disappointment. "We could have had a
double wedding!" she said half-seriously.

242

Her father laughed. "Bella and Fremont, Harriett and me?" He shook his head. "We're both too old for that. I'm sixty-three, after all, and Harriett isn't much younger."

Charlotte looked sharply at her father. His expression was bland. She wondered if he had simply lost count, or if he was consciously minimizing the difference in years between himself and Harriett. She knew her father was on the threshold of his seventieth year. She had always assumed Harriett to be about the same age she herself was. A year or so older, perhaps, although she didn't look a minute past forty.

Charlotte wondered, too, how her father would handle the marriage certificate. Harriett had been born into a community of Santee Sioux. There was no record of her parents nor her date of birth. Charlotte guessed that to satisfy the Ontario registrar general, her Sioux father would officially become a McKay. Her mother would be given whatever maiden name sprang to Joseph's mind. Her stated birthdate would likely coincide with Charlotte's own. Charlotte was aware of her father's willingness to adapt rules to circumstances. What he sought was a socially acceptable end to the six years of loneliness that had begun with the death of his second wife.

"God bless you both," said Charlotte.

Bella was married at one o'clock the following afternoon. The ceremony was scheduled to coincide with the Whitemouth train timetable, which dictated the arrival and departure of the guests from east and west, as well as the couple's honeymoon trip to Detroit. Bella wore her mother's wedding gown.

Over many hours leading up to the wedding, Charlotte had had to draw on her considerable talents as a seamstress. Bella was notably taller than Charlotte herself was, and proportionately more fully favoured. The dress was of white satin, richly trimmed in Honiton lace, with a white tulle veil. In her hands, gloved in elbow-length white kid, she carried a nosegay of spring flowers. Her three younger sisters and her cousin Margaret wore identical bridesmaids' dresses of white tarlatan. Two had pink sashes; two blue. The marriage was performed by the Reverend Charles Pitblado, rector of St. Andrew's Presbyterian Church in Winnipeg.

After the ceremony, a reception and buffet luncheon was held at the Ross house. Everyone then had to hurry, out-of-town guests and the newlywed couple as well, to catch the afternoon train to Winnipeg. Charles and his family caught a connecting train west to Brandon and home to Broadline Farm. William was anxious to attend the gala that evening for the new Canadian Pacific Railway Depot in Winnipeg. Three storeys high, of brick and stone, it replaced the simple frame building that had been Manitoba Railway Station No. 1. Charlotte had overheard her brother and his wife discussing it at the reception. Their conversation obviously had been an extension of one begun earlier.

"It will be a good party," she had heard William say. "Everyone who's anyone in Winnipeg will be there."

"Then you go," Caroline had replied.

"You're sure you don't mind?"

"Of course not. Our niece's wedding has been party enough

for me for one day." Abruptly his wife had turned away, dismissing the subject.

Bella, her bridegroom and her grandfather had rail connections to make in Winnipeg for St. Paul, Chicago and Detroit. It had been Fremont's suggestion that their honeymoon also be a homecoming, an opportunity for Bella to meet with his family and friends. Joseph would be remaining on the train for the border crossing at Detroit and the relatively short run from Windsor to London.

Charlotte and the rest of the family saw everyone off at the station. As the train pulled out, Charlotte thought of all the times that she had been the one who was leaving, and Bella the one left behind. She remembered most vividly the first time, when she had gone to Clinton to care for Mary Anne. It had been just before Bella had turned seven. Charlotte could still see her lunging towards the moving car on the Montreal station platform, shouting to her mother to take her with her. As David pulled Bella back, Charlotte could hear herself calling out to him to speak to her. He had had to speak to Bella on railway station platforms many times after that. Perhaps, Charlotte chided herself, too many times. The demands that the study and practice of medicine had made on her over the years had been heavy. Doubtless they had been equally so on the children; on Bella, the eldest, in particular. As Charlotte walked with David back to where their carriage and pair were tethered, she absently fingered a ring Fremont had given her. Before she stepped up into the phaeton, she slipped it from her finger. As she took her seat, she dropped the ring into her handbag and snapped it shut.

When Charlotte's father got off the train in London, Harriett was waiting for him. They were married within the hour by the Reverend G.R. Sanderson, rector of the Methodist Church in East London. His wife, Clara, and the church sexton served as witnesses.

The day after Bella's wedding, the smallpox that Charlotte had predicted would not stop at Rosslyn Camp broke out in two nearby settlements. There were three deaths in as many days at St. Norbert, a small community just south of Winnipeg. There were two others in St. Agathe, which lay a little farther south. In mid-April, Whitemouth was shaken by the news that a middle-aged New Brunswick man had been found dead in his room at the Syndicate Hotel. Charlotte confirmed that he had died of smallpox.

It was just before noon on the following Wednesday. David was seated at his desk in the mill office, talking with Walter Wardrop, when Charlotte entered. They both fell silent.

"One of the men was up to the house," Charlotte said to her husband. "He asked me to come down."

"Yes," said David. He gestured at his foreman. "Walter here wants to have a word with you."

Charlotte held her breath. She hoped that she knew what he was about to say. Within an hour of confirming the cause of death at the Syndicate Hotel, she had asked David to remind his young foreman of a promise he had made to give some thought to being vaccinated. This had been shortly after her return from

Rosslyn Camp. She needed someone to submit to the simple, but vital, immunization procedure to show the rest of the towns-people that there were no ill effects. She needed a Judas goat.

Her husband's foreman suited perfectly. Just going on thirty, he was both liked and respected by everyone who knew him. He was seen as a good family man, sober and dependable. These were qualities that David demanded of his mill and bush crews, his foremen, in particular. Charlotte was aware that if Walter Wardrop agreed to be vaccinated, his decision would carry a lot of weight.

"You can vaccinate me," he said.

Charlotte beamed. She did not know whether it was his friendship with David or her assurance that he and his family would be safe from smallpox that had caused him to decide in favour of the vaccination. Perhaps, she speculated, a little of both. She could not dwell on it. He still seemed apprehensive.

"You're sure there's no danger," he said. "Of my getting smallpox, I mean."

"None," said Charlotte. "The vaccine is harmless to humans. It gives you a mild case of cowpox. This makes you immune to cowpox, and smallpox too."

The young foreman looked a little sceptical. "You can do that just by scratching my arm?"

"You'll scarcely feel it. It may give a little discomfort, up to the ninth or tenth day, but that's all. I promise."

Charlotte became aware that work in the mill had stopped. About a dozen men were bunched at the open door to the office.

She caught the broad wink that her husband gave his foreman.

"The rest of the boys are here to see how Walter makes out," said David. "If he doesn't holler too loud, they've agreed to get in line."

It came to Charlotte with a rush that the two men had cooked this up between them. Not only did she have her first Whitemouth convert to vaccination, but she also had the entire crew of her husband's mill converted. She realized with a quickening pulse that their wives and children, neighbours and friends, would follow suit. She could scarcely believe it.

"Don't move, either of you!" said Charlotte. "I'll get my bag!"

She had enough vaccine on hand to do the mill crew. She would telegraph William and ask him to put whatever he had in his pharmacy on the next train and bring in more. She was confident that she would soon be immunizing not just in Whitemouth, but throughout the surrounding region as well. The thought came to Charlotte that William Hales Hingston would be proud of her.

Charlotte worked over the mill lunch break. She had vaccinated her husband's foreman first, then the men who worked under him. There were no abstainers. Feelings of uneasiness and even fear quickly gave way to confidence and bravado. There was first relief, then amusement, that the vaccination process itself was nothing more than the small scratch that Charlotte had promised. No one, beginning with their foreman, cried out in pain or fell ill with instant smallpox. The first stage of her immunization program was a success. Charlotte knew that she had only to wait now for the men to begin bringing their families to her. The rest of the community would follow. Finally, as the word got around, the homesteaders and bush workers would begin arriving at her door.

The last vaccination was done. Charlotte packed up her medical bag and walked back to the house. The men had missed most of their lunch break. David walked out onto the shop floor, where they were preparing to return to work, and gave them an extra hour. Then he asked Walter Wardrop to join him in his office. He shut the door behind them and walked to the safe behind his desk. David took the key from a drawer and bent over the safe. He reached inside and took out a bottle of Glenmorganic Scotch whiskey and two glasses. He set the glasses down on his desk. As he uncorked the bottle he grinned at his foreman.

"We'll drink to the last of the smallpox," said David. "And a good riddance to it!"

He poured a generous two fingers into both glasses. They emptied them at a swallow. David coughed appreciatively, put the cork back in the bottle and returned it to the safe.

"Not a word about this," he said. "It's one bottle the doctor doesn't know about. If she did, it would end up in her damn medicine."

Charlotte kept a flask of whiskey in her medical bag. She used it as a stimulant when a patient was in shock or suffering from exposure. The medicine David referred to was one of her own making. She administered it as a treatment for the common cold. It was a mixture of whiskey and Scott's emulsion, a popular

249

patent medicine with a cod liver oil base. She called it *Scotch emulsion.*

Charlotte and Walter Wardrop ran into each other a few days later at the post office. Standing near the doorway, out of earshot of the others who had come to pick up their mail, Charlotte addressed her husband's foreman. "How much drink did you and Mr. Ross have the day of the vaccinations? Just one, I trust."

"Drink?" echoed Walter.

From his panicked expression, Charlotte could see that she already had him in rout. "From the bottle of whiskey Mr. Ross keeps in his office safe," she said.

The young foreman capitulated. "Just one," he said.

"Good," said Charlotte. "Mr. Ross has high blood pressure. He shouldn't drink at all." She paused to let this be understood. "He can live with the occasional one," she said. "As can I."

She turned to leave. There was a hint of a smile on her lips. "Good day, Mr. Wardrop."

He opened the door for her.

"Thank you for what you did at the mill," she said.

Late in May, Charlotte learned that two important family events were to take place. One was blessed, the other historical. She realized that David and she were again expecting. If her pregnancy went full term, which would be unusual for her, she would be having their baby early in the new year. She also heard from her father that he was going to be guest of honour at the First International Railway Exposition in Chicago.

The Exposition opened on the last Friday in May. It ran for a period of one month. Its exhibits traced the history of railroading over the sixty years since George Stephenson had built the world's first steam-driven passenger train. The Rocket, which Joseph had fired as a boy of ten and a *protégé* of Stephenson's, was one of the principal attractions. As was Joseph himself, as the world's oldest living railroader.

Shortly after the Exposition ended, Joseph and Harriett moved into the house in Winnipeg. Charlotte and Harriett had liked each other from their first meeting. They seized now upon the opportunity to develop their step-family relationship and become close friends. Charlotte's father was winding down his business interests in the West. Before the Manitoba winter set in, he intended to sell the house on Logan Avenue and return to Clinton.

Harriett was a frequent guest at the Rosses'. Charlotte was a familiar figure on the train between Whitemouth and Winnipeg, and in and around the shops of Main Street and Market Square. Her Norwich canary was her travelling companion. She carried him in his lightweight japanned cage almost everywhere she went. She called him Johnny, which was short for John Bull. Sometimes it was just Charlotte and Harriett together, window-shopping. Or dropping in to have a word with Miss Beswetherick, at Alexander and Bryce. Or looking at all the beautiful things at David's cousin's, D.R. Dingwall, Jeweller. Often Caroline came with them.

Joseph and Harriett left Winnipeg in late November to live in Clinton. A few weeks later, on Christmas Day, Charlotte gave birth to a son. Had it been a girl, she had intended to name her in honour of her stepmother, Harriett. The name she chose instead was Donald McKay Ross. Donald was a Ross family name. McKay was for the surname that Harriett never had.

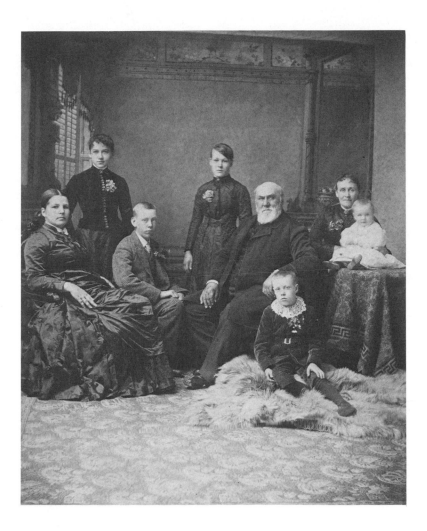

1 Charlotte and four of her children spent Christmas, 1888, at her father's house in Clinton. Seated (from left) are Harriett, Hales, Joseph Whitehead, Charlotte and Lottie. Standing are Charlotte's cousin, Alice Whitehead (left), and Carrie. Seated on the fur rug is Joseph.

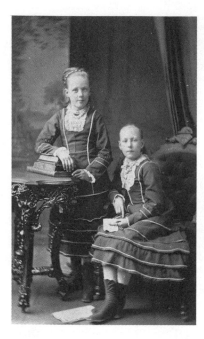 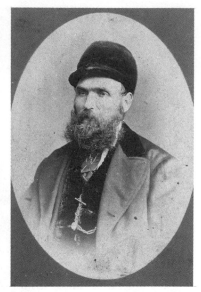

2 Charlotte, standing, with her
chronically ill elder sister, Mary Anne.

3 David Ross, Charlotte's husband,
before he emigrated from Scotland.

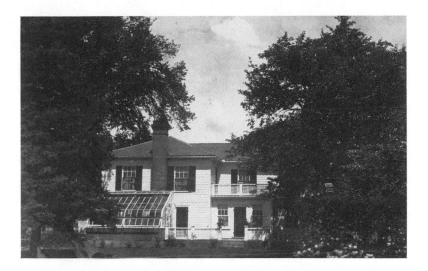

4 A stately home on three acres, the house that Charlotte grew up in has been added to and modernized over the years. It is now an apartment block at 69 Victoria Street, Clinton.

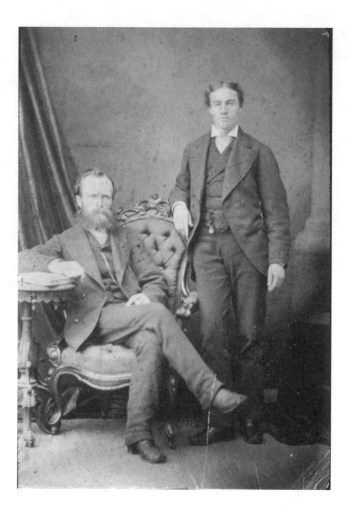

5 David Ross (seated) with his brother, Donald, during David's association with the wholesale firm of Whitehead and Ross, in Montreal.

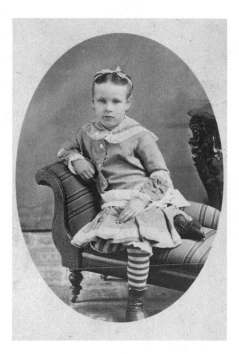

6 Caroline Cleveland (Carrie) Ross.

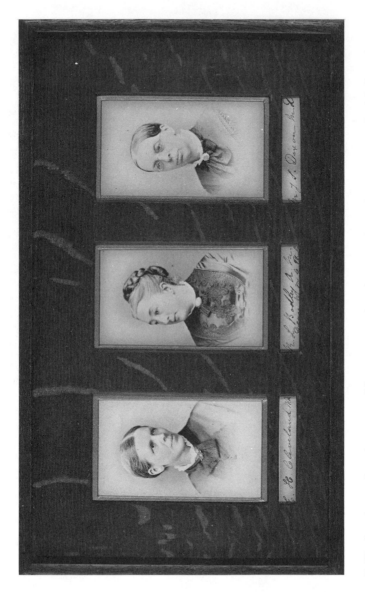

7 Charlotte hung a framed grouping of three portraits when she returned from the Woman's Medical College of Philadelphia. From left, Doctors Emeline Cleveland, Rachel Bodley and Mary Scarlett Dixon were role models to the young graduate.

8 Two pages from one of Charlotte's notebooks during her final year at the Woman's Medical College of Philadelphia.

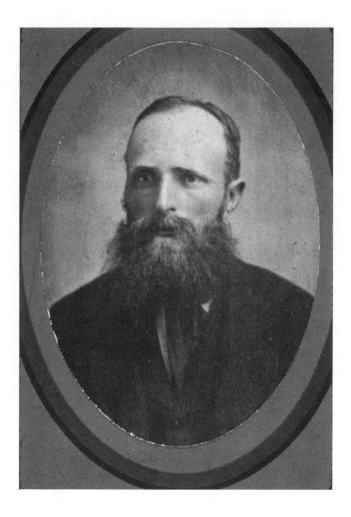

9 David, Charlotte's husband, owner of the Ross mill, in Whitemouth, Manitoba.

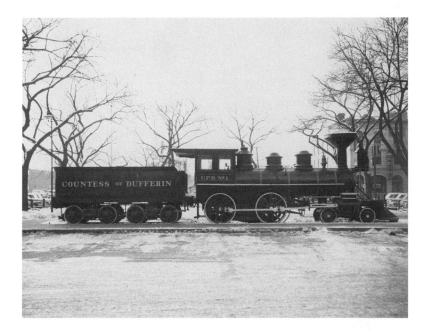

10 "The iron horse" was the term used to identify the early locomotive. This one, barged in by Charlotte's father, was the first in the West. Now moth-balled in Winnipeg, it stood for some years outside the Canadian Pacific Railway station there.

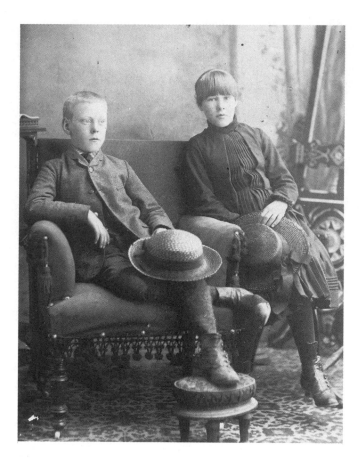

11 Hales Hingston and Mary Anne Fair (Min) Ross.

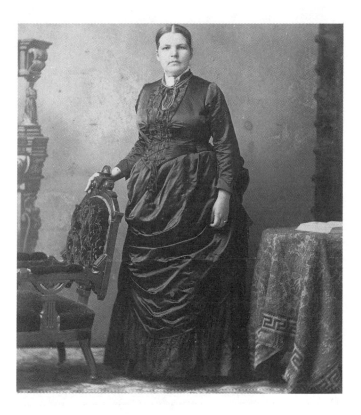

12 Harriett, Joseph Whitehead's third wife.

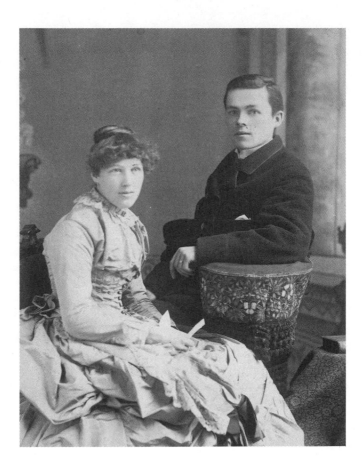

13 Min and her husband, Hope Ross. Although Hope had the same surname, he was related to his wife and her family only by marriage.

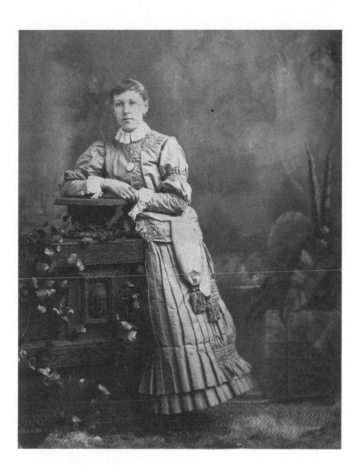

14 Catherine Laurence (Kate) Ross during a visit with American relatives in Palatka, Florida.

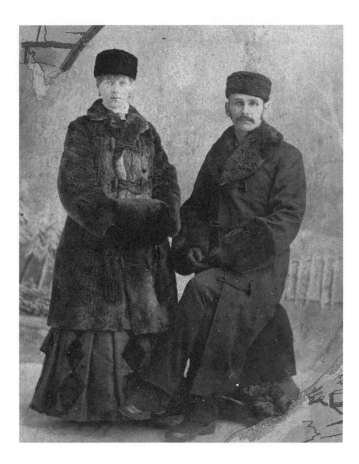

15 Kate and Peter Duncan (P.D.) McKinnon in their winter
wedding picture.

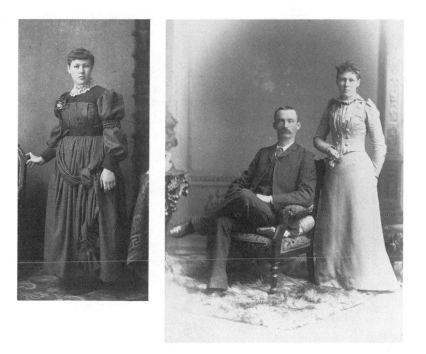

16 To finish her education, Carrie lived
a year in Clinton with her grandfather,
Joseph, and Harriett. She sent this
photograph to her mother.

17 William Barton, the railway station
agent at Whitemouth, and Carrie.

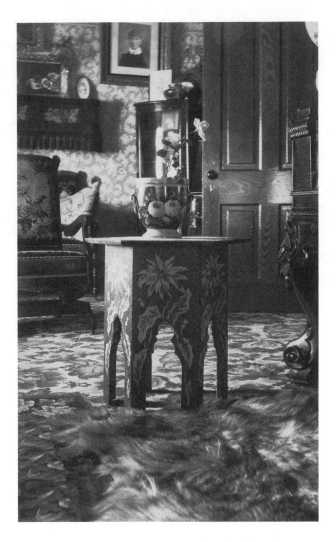

18 The parlour in the Ross house at Whitemouth.

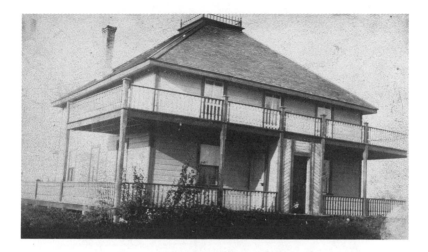

19 The frame house that replaced the original log one, Whitemouth.

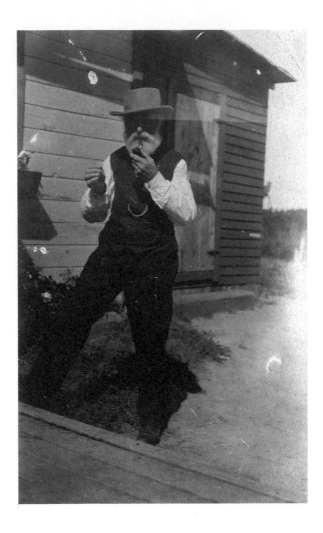

20 David, Charlotte's husband, lights up his pipe by the
summer kitchen, in Whitemouth.

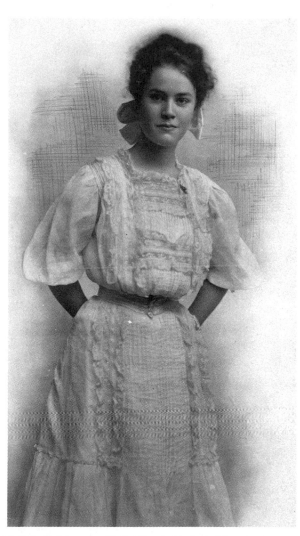

21 Isabella Margaret (Bella) Ross's daughter, Winnifred,
Charlotte's granddaughter.

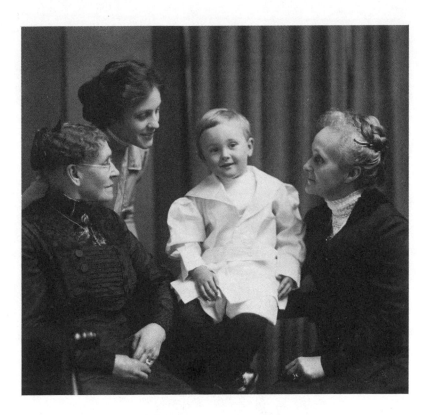

22 From left: Charlotte; Bella's daughter, Winnifred, and son; and Bella.

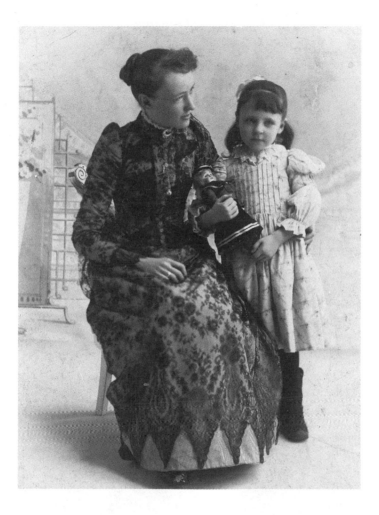

23 Min Ross with her daughter, Edith. Charlotte called her "my little
helper." Edith eventually studied medicine at the University of Manitoba and became the province's first woman anaesthetist.

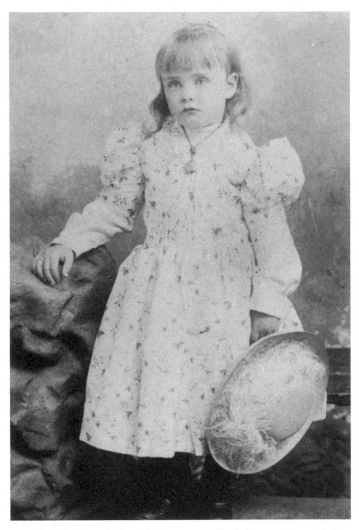

24 Lottie McKinnon Ross. Born prematurely, she was so tiny at birth that David feared she would not live, and her sisters nicknamed her "Dot." Both she and the nickname survived.

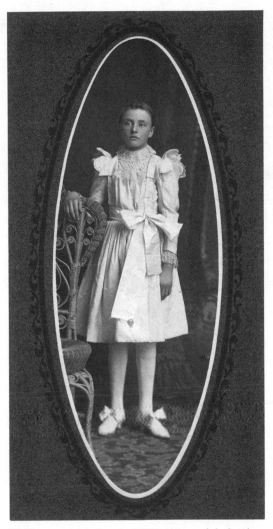

25 Dot in a party dress in 1901, one month before her thirteenth birthday.

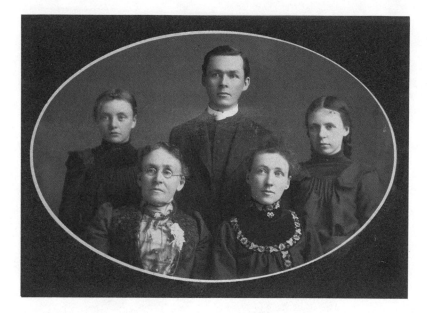

26 From left: Dot; Charlotte; Hope Ross; his wife, Min; and their daughter, Edith.

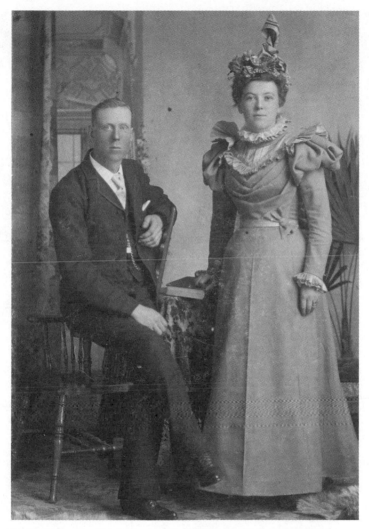

27 Hales Ross and his bride, Isabella. David gave Hales and his younger brother, Joseph, $20,000 each to invest in a lumber mill in Elkhorn, British Columbia. They moved there in 1905.

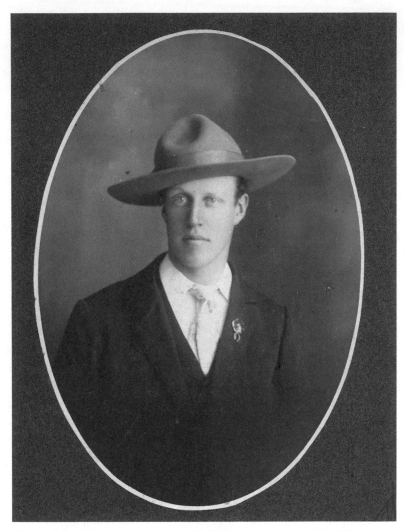

28 Joseph Ross, as co-owner with brother Hales of the lumber mill at Elkhorn.

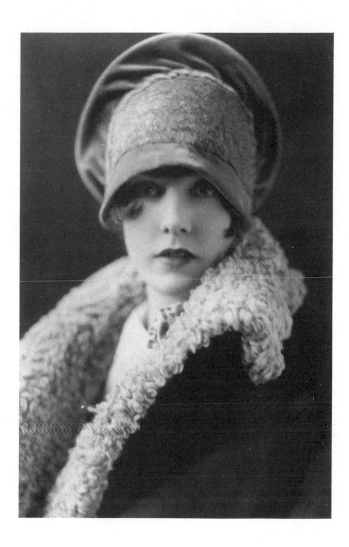

29 A generation later, in the 1930s, this was Dot's daughter, Ruth, Charlotte's granddaughter, at 17.

CHAPTER ❦ FIFTEEN

Whitemouth, Summer, 1886

*C*HARLOTTE WAS BENT OVER the rose bushes in her garden when she heard the whistled approach of the first through train from Montreal to Vancouver. It was very early. On its maiden run, the Canadian Pacific's transcontinental was chasing the sun across the evergreens and granite, around the lakes and over the rivers between Rat Portage and Whitemouth. Charlotte straightened and faced the house.

"It's coming!" she called out. "If you want to see, you'll have to hurry, everyone!"

She gathered the roses she had cut into a loose bouquet and stepped briskly around to the front. Min was the first to join her. By one hand she held Bella's two-year-old daughter, named Hanna Whitehead Wood for Bella's favourite aunt. The other clasped the hand of her own youngest brother, Donald McKay, who was six months older than Hanna. Hales and his younger brother spilled from the house with Carrie. Hales, just turned eleven, was teasing his thirteen-year-old sister about something or other until a glance from his mother put a stop to it. David came out last, stepping back to hold the door open for his eldest daughter. Bella carried her infant daughter, Winnifred, in her arms.

Over the previous few weeks, everyone had been excitedly looking forward to the arrival of the first transcontinental train. It was thought especially fitting that it would reach Winnipeg, which called itself the bull's eye of the Dominion, on Dominion Day. The cheering crowd waiting to greet the train as it crossed over the Louise Bridge was expected to be just as large as the one that had seen it off at Montreal's Dalhousie Street Station three days earlier. The train had pulled out past an honour guard of militiamen from the Victoria Rifles. It had begun its six days' run to Vancouver to a fifteen-gun salute from the Montreal Field Battery.

As Charlotte and her family watched, the train emerged from its corridor in the forest. It had a large white replica of the British Royal Crown mounted on the front of its boiler, directly above the cowcatcher. The rest of the engine, from the tops of its drive wheels to the tip of its tall smokestack, was covered with looped streamers and garlands of flowers and evergreens. Two baggage cars were coupled behind the engine. Two colonist cars came next, followed by two first-class. A dining car separated these from the two sleeping cars that made up the rear of the train.

"The Holyrood!" Hales called out, as the dining car passed below. "The Yokohama! The Honolulu!"

Charlotte thought they were odd names.

"It's the Canadian Pacific's way of selling itself as the overland route to the Orient," said David. "They're putting a third sleeping car on for passengers boarding in Winnipeg. It's named the Selkirk."

254

"Much more appropriate," said Charlotte. "Will the train stop in Whitemouth?" asked Min.

"Just briefly," said her father. "They'll want to make the best time they can to the West Coast."

A large crowd was expected at the new Whitemouth station. The Canadian Pacific had promised the world's finest sleeping-car and dining-car service. The luxuriously appointed sleeping cars had baths. The mahogany panelled dining cars with damask table cloths each boasted $3,000 worth of silver service.

"It's small wonder that people will be hoping for a close look," said Charlotte.

While she spoke, the transcontinental passed from sight. A moment later they heard it blow a fanfare on its steam whistle. The world's greatest train was announcing its approach to its first stop in the North-West. As Charlotte turned to herd the family inside for breakfast, a rose dropped from her bouquet. She stooped to retrieve it. The Yorkist roses that no one but she had thought would survive had thrived in the five years since she had planted them. She often brought bouquets of the fragrant white blossoms on her post-natal visits to new mothers. On the homesteads especially, there was little else in the house that was meant just to be beautiful.

After breakfast, Charlotte set out for a farm that was an hour away over corduroy and rutted roads through the bush northeast of Whitemouth. Before leaving the stable she smeared her team's heads with a mixture of pine tar and coal oil, against bulldog flies. Charlotte had never heard of bulldog flies before she had come to Whitemouth. She had learned in her first summer that they were a much more serious problem than the horse flies back in Clinton had been. Horses sometimes ran amok from the sheer fright and pain of an attack. Charlotte had seen them covered with bleeding sores. The pine-tar and coal-oil mixture provided some protection.

Mosquitoes, too, seemed to be both epidemic and more vampire-like than she had ever encountered elsewhere. The peat bogs and muskeg throughout the region were near-perfect breeding grounds. In the tall grass and underbrush they sometimes swarmed in clouds as big and grey as wolfskins.

David had built their house high enough on a hill to catch the river breezes, so bulldog flies and mosquitoes mercifully were not a problem for Charlotte and her family. This was not the case for homesteaders living within the still and damp enclosure of the forest. While they cleared the land with two-man bucksaws, axes and grub hoes, then drained the bogs, a ring of smudge pots was set out. These helped preserve the sanity of the homesteaders' horses and oxen, as well as their own.

Charlotte gave her team their head, letting them jog along at a leisurely gait. She looked upon it as a kind of gift to both her horses and herself in observance of a pleasant morning and the country's nineteenth birthday. There was another, more practical, reason. Her driving team was Negro and Negress, a handsome black gelding and mare that David had bought at the auction of the James McKay estate. In early spring the mare had put a hoof through a rotted timber in a log bridge. She had gone down in a panic, breaking her right foreleg. David had said she would have to be shot. Charlotte had asked that a broad, under-belly sling be rigged from the barn rafters. The mare had been hoisted to a standing position by some of the men from the mill, and Charlotte had put splints and a plaster cast on her foreleg. The break had knit, but it needed a little more time to be fully recovered.

It was for her own sake, too, that Charlotte chose to go slowly on this quiet summer morning. She believed that memories so recent that they were just drowsing should be reawakened gently. So much had happened over the past three years. There had been pleasant elements and tragic ones in about equal measure, a general prescription for life that Charlotte long before had understood and accepted.

Kate had taken a good husband in Peter Duncan McKinnon. Everyone called him plain "P.D." He was a railway worker from Broadview, a small settlement in the North-West Territories not far from the Manitoba border. They had been married at the Ross house on the Christmas Day before last. Kate had died six months later. She had succumbed quickly and unexpectedly to consumption. The same wretched condition that had claimed Mary Anne's life had shadowed her niece's lungs for most of her nineteen years and nine months.

Charlotte and David had not been by her side. At spring break-up they had left for Quebec City and the seven days' Atlantic crossing promised by Cunard's first all-steel passenger ship, the SS Servia. They had already seen David's relatives in Ross-shire and were visiting with Charlotte's in Yorkshire when they received word by undersea cable of Kate's death. Deep in her own grief, Charlotte had sat down that night and written a letter edged in black to P.D.

The day before Kate died, Caroline had given birth to a son, a brother for William Jr. They had named him Peter, for Caroline's father. All had been going well for William. He had become Whitehead and Co. and was looking at adding the second link to his chain of drugstores west.

Charles had sold Broadline Farm and had quit the land. Falling prices and an early, crop-killing frost the previous autumn had persuaded him to return to railway construction. Initially, Charlotte recalled, it had seemed like a poor choice. The country had slipped into a depression. Financing for the completion of the Canadian Pacific had faltered. It had taken the threat of a Métis uprising in the North-West Territories, and the railway's ability to get troops there quickly, to put the company back on track. Charles had won the contract to build a section along the north shore of Lake Superior.

Near the end of March, just a few days before Charlotte and David left for the British Isles, the second Métis rebellion in the North-West had begun. Louis Riel again had been the leader. Under his field commander, Gabriel Dumont, a detachment of North-West Mounted police had been defeated at Duck Lake, on the South Saskatchewan River. When Charlotte and David passed through Toronto and Montreal on their way to Quebec

City, they had seen trainloads of militiamen heading west. The fighting had ended with the defeat and capture of Riel in mid-May at Batoche, not far from where it had all started.

Charlotte and David had made the return crossing and had arrived back in Whitemouth the first week in August. Three months later, on the first Saturday in November, the last half mile of track west had been laid at Craigellachie, in the mountains of British Columbia. Louis Riel had been hanged nine days later at Regina.

Charlotte always saw these two events in a strangely personal light. Her father had played a major role in the construction of the Manitoba section of the railway that had proved so strategic militarily. Among the volunteers and the regular militia that had fought under Major General Frederick Middleton had been many young men who were her neighbours. The Reverend Charles Pitblado, who had celebrated both Bella's and Kate's weddings, had served as military chaplain with the Halifax Battalion. Her friend Father Lacombe had used his influence among the Indian tribes of the North-West Territories to dissuade all but two Cree chiefs, Big Bear and Poundmaker, from massing their braves behind the rebels.

Father Lacombe had once told Charlotte that he and another priest, Father Jean Baptiste Baudin, had witnessed the hanging of a murderer in Winnipeg. Both had wept. Charlotte thought that the priest must have wept again on the day that they hanged Louis Riel. It had been seventeen years since the Métis had rebelled against perceived injustice and flown their flag briefly over Fort Garry. While she deplored the violence, Charlotte had empathized with the Métis leader and his people.

The homestead came in sight. It lay a half mile or so ahead, over an uncertain trail through the tall grasses and small yellow sowthistle flowers of an open meadow. It was too close to the high heat of midday for the bulldog flies and mosquitoes to be at their worst. Even so, Charlotte urged her team forward. As Negro and Negress leaned into the traces, Charlotte knew that she would never lose the disturbing thought that, while Riel had acted wrongly, he had done so for the right reasons.

Charlotte tethered her team to a railing at the front of the cabin. She reached into the rear of the phaeton and lifted out a carpetbag and the bouquet of roses she had picked that morning. The family's eldest daughter opened the rough board door to her knock. Lavina was seventeen. She had four younger sisters, including the infant born three days earlier, and six brothers ranging in years from ten to nineteen.

"How is your mother today?" asked Charlotte.

"She's just fine, ma'am. She's sleeping."

Charlotte lowered her voice. "Good."

The girl's eyes were locked on the carpetbag that Charlotte set down on the planked table. Charlotte restrained a smile at her rapt curiosity. "Here," she said, giving her the bouquet. "Put these in a jar with some water for your mother."

"Dr. Ross?"

The voice came from behind a blanket hung from the ceiling to curtain off sleeping quarters in the one-room cabin. It was followed by a snuffled cry from the new baby. Charlotte pushed back the blanket and entered. The baby was making gluttonous sounds at her mother's breast. The woman lay between cotton sheets on a ticking stuffed with straw. The bedstead, the only one in the cabin, was iron. Beside it stood a simple wood cradle that the woman's husband had made for their first-born. The ten older children took down pallets at night and slept on the other side of the hanging blanket.

Charlotte knew that this was not the poorest of the families that made up her practice. They had about as much as most of the other emigrants from Europe in their first few years on their homestead. Most had arrived with no more money than it took to pay the nominal price for their land and build a rough cabin on it. Everyone including the children worked to survive. On winter nights they sat at a table by the fire and picked weed seeds from the seed grain to be planted in spring. On summer days they filled their aprons with sowthistles and grubbed for roots to burn in smudge pots while the older boys and their father worked the fields.

Lavina brought in the flowers. She had arranged them in a deep jar that served as a vase. They seemed to rouse a precious memory. The woman watched her daughter place them on a rough table by her bed. She thanked Charlotte quietly, without taking her eyes off the bouquet of white roses. The sight and scent of them seemed to mesmerize her, removing her gently to some other time and place, reminding her of some life that she had known.

Charlotte felt uncomfortably intrusive. "I brought some things," she said.

The woman nodded absently.

Charlotte crossed to the other side of the hanging blanket and opened the carpetbag. The woman's daughter followed right behind. Now Charlotte did smile, amused by the girl's growing impatience to see what she had brought with her. Charlotte took out four loaves of bread that she had baked the night before, and set them on the table. Next came a roast of beef wrapped in heavy brown paper, bought at Jackson McKinley's butcher shop. This was followed by two bags filled with potatoes, carrots, several onions and a large turnip.

"This will provide enough beef stew for the next few days," said Charlotte. "Do you know how it's made?"

The girl nodded quickly.

"I'm sure it will be a welcome change from rabbit, or whatever else you've been having."

"Rabbit and sturgeon," said the girl. "Mostly rabbit."

Charlotte reached again into the carpetbag and pulled out a bag of apples. "There's one for each of you," she said. "Ten in all. There's none for your new baby sister. She has no use for apples just yet."

Lavina smiled at this. She took one of the apples from the bag. She began polishing it on the hem of her dress, a patchwork of bleached flour sacks, sewn together and dyed.

Charlotte rummaged deeper into the carpetbag. She came up with a stack of baby's clothes. Most were from Donnie's layette, practical durables that had outlasted his infancy. Some were pretty things that she had embroidered over the winter while she prayed for another daughter. Not to replace Kate, but to fill the emptiness she had left behind. Charlotte would be forty-three in two weeks. For a few years yet she could safely bear another child.

Before Charlotte left the homestead, she made sure that the new mother was comfortable and her baby healthy. There were some women who could give birth in the morning and be back helping their husbands with the seeding or flailing that same afternoon. Charlotte had not met many. Most women needed at least a day or two to get back on their feet. She also looked to see if the woman's daughter had followed her instructions on how to go about cleaning the cabin. She noticed the two pails and cloths, still wet, standing by the woodstove beside a can of lye. The paring knife the girl had used was lying on the table.

"You did well," said Charlotte. "Germs have no place to breed in a clean house."

Charlotte clucked her team forward and started back for Whitemouth. She was grateful for the older daughter. With some of the younger homestead families, she had to roll up her sleeves and scrub down their cabins herself. When this was done, she would cook enough food to last for two or three days. Then she knew the mother would get the rest she needed and the nourishment she needed, in surroundings as aseptic as possible.

When she cleaned and cooked for these families, Charlotte seldom got home until after dark, even in the long days of summer. It was always to a dinner cooked and kept warm for her by one of her two older daughters. Because Bella's husband spent most of his time on the road, she and their two children lived with Charlotte and David. Min, who was eighteen, had a steady beau in William Barton, the station agent. Although nothing had been announced, they had an understanding. Over Easter weekend William had given Min what family and friends took for an informal engagement ring.

Another Christmas came and went before Charlotte could spend the vacation in Winnipeg that she had promised herself the previous mid-summer. As much as she longed for a lengthy stay with her two brothers and their families, it was impossible for Charlotte to take a few weeks off. She was still the only doctor practising in Whitemouth and the surrounding region. She was kept constantly busy by a burgeoning caseload of work-related accidents, illnesses and maternities among families in which ten children or more was not considered unusual. Whatever time she did not spend in actually treating patients was consumed by the distances and difficulties involved in getting to see them.

In the hiatus between late winter and early spring when no one was hurt, sick or having a baby, or seemed about to be, Charlotte made the time she needed. Apart from wishing to see William and Charles and to do the shops with Caroline and Hanna, she was concerned professionally. She had decided to meet in Winnipeg with a lawyer. It was obvious that the loosely structured nature of medical practice in the West was changing. It was now possible to obtain a doctorate in Winnipeg. The

Manitoba Medical College occupied classrooms at the corner of
Main Street and what had been the old Portage la Prairie Road,
now Portage Avenue. Its first annual commencement was to be
held within the month.

Two women doctors licensed by the Manitoba College of
Physicians and Surgeons had set up a joint practice. Originally
from Madoc, a village near Belleville, Ontario, they were a
widowed mother and her daughter. Charlotte had paid Amelia
and Lilian Yeomans a social call soon after their arrival. Amelia
had told Charlotte that her late husband had also been a doctor.
Augustus Yeomans had practised in Madoc before moving with
his wife and daughter to the United States. He had served as a
surgeon with the Army of the North during the American Civil
War. After his death, she and Lilian had enrolled in medicine at
the University of Michigan, in Ann Arbor. Her daughter had
graduated five years ago. A few months later, Lilian had fulfilled
the requirements set down by the College of Physicians and
Surgeons and had been licensed to practise in Manitoba. Amelia
had graduated the year following. She had not applied to be
licensed until two years later.

As well as the fact that she felt her doctorate was her licence
to practise, Charlotte had little in common with Amelia and
Lilian. She had always considered this a pity. When Charlotte
had called to welcome them to Winnipeg, they had sat down to
afternoon tea in their flat. Charlotte had hoped to establish a
professional relationship as well as a social one. This had not

happened. Separated by just seventy-two miles of railway track between Winnipeg and Whitemouth, she and the Yeomans were a world apart in their practice of medicine.

Charlotte gave a sideways glance as she walked past the Main Street storefront with the sign over it that read American Plumbing Company. Lettered on the door leading up to their combined offices and living quarters were the names Dr. Amelia Yeomans and Dr. Lilian B. Yeomans. It did not look like a much-travelled entry.

Charlotte had always thought this to be unfortunate but understandable. She doubted that there was one man in Winnipeg who would seek out a woman doctor. Unless, perhaps, he lay dying of the plague, and all the male doctors in town had predeceased him. As well, there was still prejudice against women doctors by some women, or by their fathers and husbands, which amounted to the same thing. Although they sometimes treated the diseases of women and children, the Yeomans practised medicine primarily as midwives.

Charlotte soon realized that this did not seem to bother them. Both mother and daughter managed to keep busy in other ways. Amelia played a prominent role in the Women's Christian Temperance Union. She and Lilian were dedicated to closing down Winnipeg's saloons and bawdy houses, cleaning up its jails, and campaigning for the vote for women. They were full-time suffragettes. While Charlotte approved of their objectives, her busy general practice and family of eight left her little time for causes.

As she continued up Main Street, Charlotte made a mental note to pay her respects to Amelia and Lilian within the next day or two. First she wanted to get her legal business out of the way. She was aloofly aware that she was being noticed. She always turned heads when she came to Winnipeg. In the summer, people looked twice at the John Bull canary she carried in its handsome ebony cage. On a day like this, cold enough for a fur coat, Charlotte's caught their eye.

The coat was one of a kind. She had had it custom-made by Edgar Dechêne, Quebec City's most fashionable furrier, while she and David were visiting overseas. The wild-mink skins had been given to her by her Indian patients. Since they had already been docked for the treaty doctor, Charlotte refused to let them pay her. The skins were gifts. She had designed the coat herself. Mr. Dechêne at first had refused to make it because it had sleeves. Ladies who wore fine furs, he had argued, especially those from the House of Dechêne, did not have to use their arms. Gentlemen escorts and servants opened doors for them and carried their parcels.

Ladies who harnessed horses to sleighs, and dug themselves out of snowdrifts, Charlotte had countered, did indeed use their arms. She wanted a coat that didn't look like a buffalo robe. Something chic that she could wear on her winter rounds that would keep her warm. Mr. Dechêne had finally thrown up his arms and made the coat, but he did it under protest. No one in the fashionable East, or anywhere else, had ever seen a mink coat like it.

It was a short walk from the storefront where the Yeomans practised to Aikins, Culver and Hamilton, Barristers and Solicitors. Their offices occupied the second floor of the Imperial Bank Building, just two blocks north on Main Street. Charlotte entered the foyer and took the stairs past a brass wall plaque that bore the firm's name. The senior partner had been Charlotte's father's lawyer in Winnipeg. He had also handled all the Canadian Pacific Railway's litigation in the Midwest.

James Aikins rose as Charlotte entered. "Dr. Ross." He came from behind his desk and took her hand before helping her off with her coat. "This is indeed a pleasure." He went back to his desk and opened the file that lay on it.

"I have studied your letter," he said. "You are requesting that we petition the government to allow you to practise medicine, surgery and midwifery in this province."

Charlotte nodded.

"You base this request on the doctorate awarded you by the Woman's Medical College of Pennsylvania, an internationally recognized school of medicine. Also on your twelve years as a respected medical practitioner, both in Quebec and here in Manitoba." He studied her a moment. "Tell me. Why have you chosen to petition at this time? Why not when you first arrived?"

"There was no need then."

"And there is now?"

Charlotte nodded. "For two reasons. The College of Physicians and Surgeons is about to redouble its efforts against anyone who practises unlicensed. I have learned that Dr. Kerr, the dean of the Manitoba Medical College, is calling on Dr. Gray, the registrar for the Physicians and Surgeons, to prosecute more actively."

William had told Charlotte this over dinner with Caroline the previous evening. It had been the prime topic of discussion, all of it favourable, among the doctors who came to his pharmacy.

"My second reason," said Charlotte, "is the boundary dispute between Manitoba and Ontario. If Whitemouth becomes part of Ontario, my position will be even less tenable than it is now. Licensed or not, I am the only doctor in the region. This, coupled with my credentials and my experience, gives me leverage here in Manitoba. I would have none whatsoever with the Ontario College of Physicians and Surgeons."

The border dispute between Manitoba and Ontario was entering its fourteenth year. It was still uncertain on which side the Whitemouth region, including the town itself, might fall.

The lawyer was thoughtful for a moment. "If yours was the only licensing petition before the Legislative Assembly, I would not be concerned. On its own, it would doubtless be given special consideration. The problem is, there will be others."

"I don't understand."

"I made some enquiries. There will be ladies who practise as midwives petitioning to be licensed. None, of course, has your professional credentials. But the members feel that they can't make an exception of one and not another."

Charlotte had not been aware of this new problem. "What do you advise, Mr. Aikins?"

The lawyer smiled reassuringly. "I advise you not to be concerned. Let me see what I can do."

Charlotte got up to go. "Then I'll leave it in your hands."

"Your father was my friend as well as a valued client over his time in Winnipeg. I trust he's well?"

"And busy," said Charlotte. "Father is running for mayor of Clinton."

The lawyer arched his eyebrows. "Mr. Whitehead is not a young man."

"Seventy-two this year," said Charlotte.

Two weeks later, Charlotte returned home to a surprise announcement from her daughter Min. Looking back on it, she realized that there had been no warning signs. Except, of course, the realization that over the past while William Barton had not been seen around the house as often as usual.

Min had a new beau. His name was Hope Ross. Although he had the same surname as Min, they were not related. A little less than three years earlier, the Presbyterian Church in Canada had established a number of mission field stations in Manitoba. Whitemouth was one of them. The young student missionary from Walkerton, Ontario, was among those assigned on weekends to conduct Sunday services at Ross Presbyterian Church. Arriving by train early on Saturdays, they stayed over as guests at the Ross house until their return to Winnipeg on Sunday evenings.

After dinner on the last Sunday in May, Hope asked David's permission to marry his daughter. He had proposed to Min that morning after church, as they strolled along the riverbank by the mill. David was pleased to give them his blessing. It had bothered him that Min might marry the station agent. William Barton, perish the thought of having one for a son-in-law, was a Conservative.

The wedding was set for the first week in October. A few days after the engagement was announced, Charlotte stopped by the railway station. From the morning that they had pumped the handcar together, over the months that he had been courting her daughter, Charlotte had grown to like young Barton. She wanted him to know this. Recessed in her mind was the thought that while Carrie was just fourteen, there was still the chance that she might one day have William Barton for a son-in-law. That evening, Charlotte told Min that she had seen her daughter's former beau and that he was hurting. Min said that she knew this. They had parted friends, and he had refused to take back the ring her had given her. Min said she didn't feel right about keeping it. She also felt that Hope might find it objectionable. Over Charlotte's own objections, she gave her mother the ring.

As she prepared for bed, Charlotte took a small velvet box from her bureau. Inside was the ring that Bella's husband had given Charlotte when he was courting her daughter. Over the past while, her son-in-law had been even more of a stranger than before. He was spending weeks on end on the road, away from his wife and two daughters. Charlotte placed the ring Barton had given Min beside it. David was already in bed. He turned over restlessly and watched his wife for a moment. She was standing quite still, looking down at the open box in her hand.

"It's getting late," said David.

Charlotte snapped the box shut and placed it in the drawer. She cupped her hand over the lamp chimney and blew out the flame. David reached for her hand as she got under the bedclothes.

"What were you doing?" he asked.

"I was putting away the 'unhappiness rings,'" said Charlotte.

She soon found that William had been right about the pressure being brought to bear on unlicensed medical practitioners by the College of Physicians and Surgeons. Mrs. Annie Power was arrested. She was found guilty of practising illegally, fined and ordered by the court to cease practising under pain of further prosecutions and penalties.

At the beginning of June, a paper was presented to the Legislative Assembly petitioning that Mrs. Power be granted a special licence to practise. It bore the signatures of fifty Winnipeg matrons, all of whom she had delivered of babies. By the end of the month, Mrs. Joseph Williams and Miss Amy Porter had also filed petitions endorsed by supporters.

Min was married on the first Monday in October, two weeks before her twentieth birthday. Like both sisters before her, she wore her mother's wedding gown. The couple's vows were heard by the Reverend D.B. Whimster of the Presbyterian Home Mission Committee, Hope's superiors in Winnipeg. A family reception followed.

Joseph had arrived with Harriett a few days early for his granddaughter's wedding. Charlotte's father was in fine form at the reception. He was obviously enjoying his modest celebrity as the newly elected mayor of Clinton. He was quick to admit that his wife had been a big help to him. It did not surprise Charlotte that in the four years that she had been in Clinton, Harriett had become known for her work among the town's poor and physically handicapped. Joseph was talking of erecting a building in Clinton and naming it the McKay Block in his wife's honour.

Charlotte's brothers and their families had arrived by train on the morning of the wedding. Charlotte realized that all was not well with William and Caroline. William was noncommittal to Charles's casual enquiry into how his drug business was doing. He was not at all his usual brashly confident self. Caroline, too, seemed withdrawn. It was nothing that they said that Charlotte found disturbing. It was more what was left unsaid.

Min and Hope drove off in the wedding present that Charlotte and David had given them. It was a blood gelding hitched to a convertible black buggy. David had ordered it from Christopher Montgomery's carriage works in Winnipeg. He had kept the horse stabled with his mill horses and the buggy hidden in the wagon shed until just after the wedding ceremony. The gift was something that the newlyweds could scarcely do without. Hope had been assigned to Clear Springs, a mission field station like Whitemouth, some distance southeast of Winnipeg.

In mid-November Charlotte paid a return visit to her lawyer in response to a letter that James Aikins had sent her. He wished to tell her what he was doing on her behalf and there were some relevant papers for her to sign.

"Three ladies practising midwifery petitioned the Legislative Assembly over the summer," he said. "All three petitions were well-supported with testimonials to character and professional competence. All three were rejected." He held up a newspaper clipping. "I assume that you've seen this?"

"I have," said Charlotte.

The clipping was a *Free Press* report on the dean's address to students at the start of the fifth annual session of the Manitoba Medical College. Dr. James Kerr had praised the College of Physicians and Surgeons for its determined campaign against illegal practitioners. He had noted that over the past while there had been nine prosecutions and eight convictions.

"It is William Luxton's editorial comment that disturbs me," said the lawyer. He read aloud: "'The general result of these prosecutions is that the Province has been pretty well rid of that class of charlatans.'" He paused. "Mr. Luxton's opinion as a newspaper editor is of no consequence," he said. "His opinion as a member of the Legislature is."

The editor of *The Daily Free Press* had been re-elected the previous December.

"Mr. Luxton could be a problem," said Aikins.

He explained that the strategy he planned was not simply to petition. This had already been tried in the three previous instances he had cited and had failed. Instead, they would seek to have a private member's bill passed. Thomas Smith, an English immigrant-farmer who sat as the Independent member for Springfield, had already been approached. He had agreed to introduce the bill.

"Express my gratitude to Mr. Smith," said Charlotte. She prepared to leave. "How soon will all this be done with?"

"Notice will appear in the *Manitoba Gazette* next month," said Aikins. "It will be heard near the end of the next session; I would think the last week in April or the first in May."

Charlotte had little time over the next few weeks to speculate on her action before the Legislature. She was much too busy with her practice. After her meeting with Aikins, she spent a few more days in Winnipeg, Christmas shopping and visiting with Hanna and her family at their house on Laura Street. Charles was not there. He was engaged in railway construction on the prairies west of Winnipeg. While the main artery east to west was completed, there were still hundreds of miles of track to be laid connecting with communities to the north and south.

As Charlotte had suspected, William's drug business was suffering serious reverses. There seemed to be no good reason.

She was both concerned and puzzled by her sister-in-law's suggestion that it had something to do with problems of his own
making. Caroline would say no more. They had moved from their
Garry Street house to a less comfortable but more economical
apartment in Westminster Flats, on Donald Street.

Caroline was keeping her two children under house quaran-
tine against scarlet fever. She was not the only one among
Winnipeg mothers. Peter was just a few months past his second
birthday, William Jr. would not be seven for another three weeks,
and both were young enough to be especially susceptible. So
many people had come down with the disease in Winnipeg that
it was being considered epidemic. Charlotte agreed with Caroline
that she should take every reasonable precaution. Particularly
among children, scarlet fever frequently proved fatal.

Charlotte returned to Whitemouth the next day. The following morning she was asked to see a sick child at a homestead some
distance from town. A few days earlier, the boy's mother told her,
he had become tired and irritable. He had developed a fever and
a sore throat. The previous night he had begun throwing up. His
father had gone for Charlotte.

She felt the child's skin. It was hot and dry. She lifted his arm.
Bright red spots had already begun to break out in the creases of
his armpits. Soon they would cover his body. She asked the boy
to open his mouth wide and say "ahhh." His throat was raw. He
already had what she recognized as strawberry tongue. In a few
days it would be a bright red.

There were six children. The family of German immigrants

lived in a two-room cabin. The sick child could not be kept away from the others. Charlotte realized that it was probably too late anyway. The disease was already well into the incubation period. Scarlet fever was unpredictable. One or more of the other children might get it. Or just a sore throat. Or not sick at all. She got the boy's mother to heat a pail of water on the cookstove and gave him a tepid bath. Then she dusted him with boric powder. She gave him a little salicylic acid in water for his sore throat and to help bring down the fever. She left a supply of boric and salicylic powders with instructions that the treatment be repeated every four hours.

Charlotte promised to return the next morning. As she was leaving, she advised the boy's mother and father to hope for the best and pray. So much of her practice, she was acutely aware, was rooted in this prescription. Hope and prayer. She recognized them as her two most efficacious medicaments.

Throughout December, Charlotte's caseload of families with scarlet fever reached epidemic proportions. It was as though rural Manitoba were a blotter, soaking up the quick scarlet stain that had spilled over from Winnipeg. It was sometimes just as swift to kill.

On Christmas Eve the disease claimed the life of a young girl in Meadow Lea, a small farming community on the Canadian Pacific's main line to the northwest. It had taken her father several hours to go by horse and buggy from their farm to the railway station to telegraph Winnipeg for a doctor. His daughter was dead on his return.

In the last week in January, Charlotte's own youngest son took sick. Donald McKay did not have scarlet fever. He had fallen seriously ill with diphtheria.

CHAPTER SIXTEEN

Whitemouth, Winter, 1888

CHARLOTTE SPENT THE NIGHT fitfully, nodding in a rocking chair by Donnie's bed. She came slowly awake now, blinking in the early morning sunshine that filled the window, pulling her knitted shawl more closely around her shoulders.

She leaned forward and put the back of her hand to her son's brow. His fever had subsided a little. She brushed aside a damp wisp of his hair with the tips of her fingers. She leaned closer and kissed his cheek.

"God bless you," she said aloud.

Charlotte got up and walked to the bedroom window. It was beginning to melt outside, a strange thing to happen at this time of year. Since she had come to Whitemouth, she could not remember another day in February that had promised to be so unseasonably warm. She walked to the kitchen. While she was brewing tea on the back of the cookstove, her husband entered.

"How is the boy?" he asked.

"No different," said Charlotte. "He's still in a coma."

David was hesitant. "You're going to stay with him?"

"I can't." Charlotte filled two cups. "A baby is calling out to me." She sat down at the table. "I can always hear them calling when their time is near." She smiled slightly. "At least, I always feel I can."

David sat down opposite her. He put a little milk in both their cups. "I wish you'd stay," he said.

Charlotte shook her head. "I've done all I can for Donnie," she said. "Now I have to do for someone else's child."

"When will you go?"

"Soon. I expect the mother will be going into labour at any time. Her husband or one of the boys will come."

They sat in silence, sipping their tea, listening to the laboured sounds of their son's breathing. After a while, there was a knock at the door.

"That will be the husband now," said Charlotte.

She got up from the table and left the room. She picked up her fur coat and her medical bag from where she had put them on a chair by the front door. Without looking back, Charlotte went to answer the call of the unborn child.

POSTSCRIPT

LTHOUGH DONALD MCKAY did not regain consciousness, Charlotte was at his bedside at the time of his death. He died late in the day on Saturday, February 18, after Charlotte had delivered the expectant mother of a daughter and returned home. Donnie was four years, two months.

Bella's elder daughter also caught diphtheria and died seventeen days later, on Sunday, March 4. Hanna was three years, nine months.

In mid-May, William Luxton opposed on principle the second reading of Bill 58 in the Legislative Assembly. The bill, legislating Charlotte the right to practise in Manitoba, was rejected.

Less than two weeks later, on Monday, May 28, Charlotte gave birth to a girl. She christened her Lottie McKinnon Ross, an abbreviation of her own name coupled with the surname of her deceased daughter's husband, P.D.

His dream of a chain of drugstores in the West ended, William left Winnipeg that same year with his wife and two sons. They moved first to Northport, Long Island, then back to

Montreal, where they eventually separated. William returned to Winnipeg in 1900, and worked as a pharmacist. He died alone three years later, in St. Boniface Hospital, from meningitis.

Charles continued in railway construction with the Canadian Pacific Railway. He and Hanna returned to live in Brandon, where they became prominent members of the community, she for her volunteer work with the Ladies Auxilliary of Brandon General Hospital, he as president of the Board of Governors.

Bella moved to Kansas City, Missouri, with her husband and daughter, Winnifred. Soon after, she and Fremont separated. Bella and Winnifred went to California, where Bella converted to Christian Science. She later became a reader in a Christian Science church.

Carrie married her sister Min's old beau, William Barton, in 1892.

In January of the following year, just months after Joseph had built and named the McKay Block in Clinton in her honour, his wife died following an unexplained period of feeling unwell. *The New Era* editorialized its surprise at her "unexpected" death. She was buried beneath a marker that reads simply "Harriett." In November, Joseph took their twenty-seven-year-old housekeeper, Catherine Little, for his fourth wife. A few weeks later, he wrote Charlotte that he was becoming progressively ill, much as Harriett had. A second letter begged her to come quickly to Clinton. Charlotte arrived shortly before her father died. On his deathbed he told her that he believed both Harriett and he had been given arsenic. Joseph died on March 12, 1894, just four months and four days after his wedding day. While Charlotte could not find signs of anything as obvious as arsenic, she never lost the suspicion that her father, and probably Harriett, had been poisoned.

William Hales Hingston was knighted by Queen Victoria in 1895 for his work both in preventive medicine and innovative surgical procedures. The following year, Sir William was appointed to the Senate in Ottawa.

Two years of failing health led to David's death, at seventy-eight, on August 15, 1912. Charlotte retired from practice soon after. She left Whitemouth and took up residence at 112 Lenore Street in Winnipeg.

Charlotte died on Monday, February 21, 1916, in her seventy-third year. She had practised medicine in Whitemouth for a quarter of a century after the Legislative Assembly rejected her bid to have her right to practise legislated. She was never prosecuted.

INDEX

abortion (*see* miscarriage)

abuse by male students 85, 104, 126, 128

Aikins, Culver and Hamilton, Barristers and Solicitors, Winnipeg 268

Aikins, James 268, 274

Albani, Madam (*see* Lajeunesse, Marie Louise Emma Cecile)

alcoholism 139

Alexander and Bryce, Winnipeg 179, 203, 251

Alexandria, Ontario 70

American Civil War 79, 81, 265

amputation 231

anaesthetic 231

Anatomy, Gray's 36

Ann Arbor, Michigan 265

arsenic 282

Assiniboine Bridge, Winnipeg 160, 175

Assiniboine River 160, 175, 211

autumnal fever (*see* typhoid fever)

Ayr, Sarah 202

Balmoral Street, Montreal 144

Bandon, Ontario 141

Bandon River 178

Barton, William Henry 231, 270, 271, 282

Baudin, Father Jean Baptiste 259

Belleville, Ontario 265

Beswetherick, Miss 179, 203, 251

Bill 58, Legislative Assembly, Manitoba 268, 281

Birch Island, Manitoba 175

Blackwood, Lord Frederick Temple, Earl of Dufferin (*see* Lord Dufferin)

Blackwell, Dr. Elizabeth 39

Bleury Street, Montreal 144

Blyth, Ontario 10, 147, 160

Bonsecours Market, Montreal 117

boric powder 124, 277

Bow River (Alberta), North-West Territory 228

Brandon, Manitoba 176, 211, 244, 282

Brandon General Hospital 282

British North America 13

Broadline Farm, Brandon 212, 244, 258

Broadview (Saskatchewan), North-West Territory 257

Buffalo, Brantford and Goderich Railroad 8, 109

Burns, Reverend Dr. Robert 109

Calgary (*see* Fort Calgary)

Campbell, Dr. Francis H. 131

Campbell, Sir John, Marquess of Lorne 235

Canada Day (*see* Dominion Day)

Canadian Illustrated News, The 26

Canadian Medical Association 27, 212, 213

Canadian Pacific Hotel, Whitemouth 219

Canadian Pacific Railway: chaplain 216;
   Contract No. 1, Land Department 211;

285